CPT Han
Psychiatrists

Second Edition

CPT Handbook for Psychiatrists

Second Edition

Chester W. Schmidt, Jr., M.D.
Department of Psychiatry
Johns Hopkins Bayview Medical Center
Baltimore, Maryland

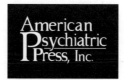

American Psychiatric Press, Inc.

Washington, DC
London, England

Contents

Preface   vii

CHAPTER 1
Introduction   1

CHAPTER 2
Basics of CPT   5

CHAPTER 3
Codes for Psychiatric Services   15

CHAPTER 4
Evaluation and Management Services   35

CHAPTER 5
Health Insurance Issues   51

CHAPTER 6
Medicare   63

CHAPTER 7
Documentation   77

CHAPTER 8
Putting It All Together for Accurate Coding   101

APPENDIX 1
Medicare Part B Carriers   115

APPENDIX 2
Vignettes for New Psychotherapy Codes   123

APPENDIX 3
**Health Care Financing Administration
Regional Offices**   137

References   141
Index   143

Preface

The second edition of this handbook, as did the first, grew out of my role on the Work Group on Codes and Reimbursements of the American Psychiatric Association (APA). The Work Group was created 8 years ago by Paul J. Fink, M.D., in part as a response to allegations of fraud brought against several departments of psychiatry. As this edition of the handbook is being written, the Health Care Financing Administration (HCFA) and the Justice Department are auditing medical schools (including departments of psychiatry) for their coding and billing practices. Several medical schools have already been penalized tens of millions of dollars as a result of the audits. Individual practitioners also have been audited, some have been fined, and some have gone to jail because of billing and coding practices.

The mission of the Work Group is to monitor and update the section of the *Physicians' Current Procedural Terminology* (CPT) manual that principally serves psychiatric practitioners and to educate the membership of the APA about coding procedures. The Work Group sponsors workshops and courses at the annual APA meeting and the Institute on Psychiatric Services. Members of the Work Group have given lectures and workshops in most of the district branches across the country and more recently are providing consultative services to hospitals, clinics, and individual practitioners through the APA Consultation Service. At every presentation, members want to know about the technical aspects of coding and the relationship between coding and reimbursement. The needs of the practitioners, expressed through their questions about coding, gave rise to the first edition of this handbook, and their needs continue to provide the basic framework for this edition.

Chapters 1 and 2 of the handbook provide basic background about CPT coding and an explanation of the format of the CPT manual and CPT Committee procedures. Chapter 3 describes in detail the psychiatric evaluation and therapeutic procedure codes. Chapter 4 describes the evaluation and management service codes. Chapters 5 and 6 focus on third-party carrier issues and the Medicare physician reimbursement system. Chapter 7 has been enhanced to cover the new documentation requirements sponsored by the American Medical Association and HCFA. Chapter 8 is a summary of the issues facing the practitioner and offers pearls of wisdom for sharpening the practitioner's ability to cope with the practical realities of coding.

The principal limitation of this handbook is that the field continues to move rapidly, and changes in documentation are occurring so quickly that certain content of the handbook is soon outdated. Despite these limitations, the expectation is that the content of this edition will enhance practitioners' knowledge of the business aspects of their practice.

This handbook could not have been possible without the Work Group on Codes and Reimbursements. Several members of the Work Group deserve particular acknowledgment for their contributions: Tracy Gordy, M.D., Ed Gordon, M.D., Bill Ayres, M.D., Melodie Morgan-Minott, M.D., David Berland, M.D., James Margolis, M.D., and Frank Rafferty, M.D. The Work Group is totally dependent on and grateful for staff support from Katherine Moore from the Office of Economic Affairs and Practice Management. Last but not least, the manuscript for this edition is due to the hard work and skill of my secretary, Sharon Greason.

CHAPTER 1

Introduction

The climate for practicing medicine and psychiatry has changed dramatically in the last decade. The introduction of the Resource-Based Relative Value Scale (RBRVS) for reimbursement of physicians by the Health Care Financing Administration (HCFA) and the effects of managed care have forever changed the business aspects of the practice of medicine. The business details of practice, such as coding, billing, completing insurance forms, and documenting services, are critical aspects of practice that have become increasingly burdensome. Procedural coding, such as diagnostic coding, is a necessary, permanent component of billing and collection activities. Coding errors often lead to rejection of insurance forms, delaying reimbursement. More importantly, errors may trigger audits by third-party payers, leading to allegations of abusive or fraudulent billing.

The practice of psychiatry now includes more treatment modalities and sites of service than ever, and the number of codes available for denoting psychiatric services has increased, thereby increasing the probability of coding disputes with third-party payers. Third-party payers have increased the requirements for documenting the services coded. The cumulative effects of all of these changes require a sophisticated knowledge of procedural coding. The American Psychiatric Association (APA) has always recognized the importance of procedural coding. In conjunction with the American Medical Association (AMA), the APA published two editions of *Procedural Terminology for Psychiatrists* (1975 and 1980). Before creating the Work Group on Codes and Reimbursements, the APA had a committee on *Physicians' Current Procedural Terminology* (CPT) coding, which was discharged and its responsibilities assumed by the Work Group. Two years ago, the Work Group was assigned permanent committee status on the Council of Economic Affairs. The APA has always had one of its members serve on the Advisory Committee to the AMA CPT Editorial Panel, and for the last 6 years, the Editorial Panel has included a psychiatrist, Tracy Gordy, M.D. The American Academy of Child and Adolescent Psychiatry also has a committee member who serves on the AMA CPT Editorial Advisory Committee.

Over the 8 years of its existence, the Work Group has identified many coding problems and issues for institutions and practitioners alike. Many practitioners unfortunately possess limited knowledge about coding. Add to the lack of knowledge rapid changes in coding practices (i.e., the introduction in 1992 of an entirely new set of evaluation and management [E/M] codes, the RBRVS payment system, the 5-year update of RBRVS, changing documentation requirements, and different payment policies of payers) and the scene is set for confusion at best, catastrophe at worst. To add to the practitioner's burden, one of the most startling discoveries of the Work Group was that the Medicare system, supposedly a national system governed by a uniform set of regulations and administered locally by third-party intermediaries, permits significant latitude to the intermediaries in interpreting the regulations. As a consequence, many practitioners are subject to idiosyncratic, arbitrary rules and payment policies of the local intermediaries. Many commercial insurance companies are following the lead of HCFA and have adopted or are in the process of adopting the RBRVS system for reimbursement of physicians, including the associated documentation requirements. Requiring documentation for clinical practice permits increased payer control of medical expenditures, affecting both patients and providers.

Increasingly, the only health services reimbursed by HCFA and commercial payers are those delivered by practitioners face-to-face with the patient. Work such as reviewing records, writing medical notes, reviewing test results, telephone calls, and case management, all vital clinical services not provided face-to-face with the patient, is supposedly "comprehended" in pre- and postservice time of the services and procedures defined by CPT and the RBRVS system. The combined system of codes, Relative Value Units (RVUs), and documentation requirements is easily monitored by the payers, and outlier practitioners can be quickly identified.

There are coding issues and problems even for managed care. The discounted fee schedules offered by commercial carriers and behavioral health carve-out companies often require using codes that vary from those in the instructions of the CPT manual. As a consequence, the practitioner must track the payment policies and code usage for each patient's insurance coverage. Although coding issues should be moot under a capitated method of payment, coding continues to be important because the distribution of the capitation to physician providers is increasingly being linked to the RVUs of the RBRVS system as a means to account for providing professional services. Solo practitioners are less affected by these issues than are physicians who practice in single-specialty or multispecialty groups.

Historically, psychiatric services were "bundled" into relatively few procedural codes. Bundling can be illustrated by reviewing the descriptor for individual medical psychotherapy (code **90841**) in CPT 97. The descriptor reads: "Individual medical psychotherapy by a physician, with continuing medical diagnostic evaluation and drug management when indicated. . . . " (American Medical Association 1996b, p. 344). The descriptor includes three services: psychotherapy, evaluation, and drug management. With the publication of CPT '98 (American Medical Association 1997), the descriptors for individual psychotherapy differentiate psychotherapy with and without E/M services, thereby beginning the process of unbundling some psychiatric services (see Chapter 3).

For better or worse, the practitioner today is confined to using a limited number of codes for psychiatric services, certain E/M codes, and a few related service codes. This handbook has been developed to help the practitioner become an expert in all aspects of procedural coding so that services are appropriately reimbursed and coding is accurate, which will eliminate, it is hoped, coding errors that lead to audits. To become an expert, the practitioner must carefully read all the relevant sections of the *Physicians' Current Procedural Terminology* each year and use this handbook as a guide to selecting appropriate codes and levels of service.

CHAPTER 2

Basics of CPT

History

Physicians' Current Procedural Terminology (CPT) was developed and first published by the American Medical Association (AMA) in 1966. The manual is a listing of descriptive terms and identifying codes for reporting medical services and procedures. The purpose of the coding system is to provide a uniform language that accurately describes medical, surgical, and diagnostic services, thus providing an effective means of communication among providers, patients, and third-party payers. The specific goals of the manual are to facilitate communication of accurate information on procedures and services to agencies concerned with claims processing, to provide the basis for a computer-based system for the evaluation of operative and diagnostic procedures, and to contribute basic information for actuarial and statistical purposes. Following the 1966 edition, three more editions were published (1970, 1973, and 1977). CPT is currently in its fourth edition and is updated annually.

In 1983, CPT was adopted as part of the Health Care Financing Administration's (HCFA's) common procedure coding system, providing the basis for reporting medical services in both the Medicare and Medicaid programs. In addition, CPT is used exclusively by most private health insurance companies. A 1987 study conducted by the AMA indicated that more than 95% of practicing physicians used CPT in their office practices. In 1975 and in 1980, the American Psychiatric Association (APA) and the AMA jointly published editions of *Procedural Terminology for Psychiatrists*. These publications were intended to serve as mini CPTs for psychiatrists, but they are no longer supported or published by the AMA and APA.

AMA CPT Editorial Panel

The responsibility for updating CPT rests with the AMA CPT Editorial Panel, composed of 15 physicians and 1 doctor of podiatric medicine. Ten physicians are nominated by the AMA, the AMA appoints the chair, and one each is nominated by the American Hospital Association, the Blue Cross/Blue Shield Association, the Health Insurance Association of America, the AMA Healthcare Professionals Advisory Committee, and HCFA. In 1983, the AMA and the U.S. Department of Health and Human Services developed an agreement that stipulated that this panel of physicians has the sole authority to revise, update, or modify CPT. No psychiatrist was a member of the CPT Editorial Panel until 1991.

CPT Advisory Committee

The CPT Editorial Panel is supported in its work by the CPT Advisory Committee, composed of practicing physicians nominated by the national medical specialty societies represented in the AMA House of Delegates. The CPT Advisory Committee now has 80 members, including a representative from the APA and one from the American Academy of Child and Adolescent Psychiatry. The primary purpose of the Advisory Committee is to serve as a technical resource to the CPT Editorial Panel. The full committee meets annually, but from time to time work groups are formed to address specific tasks on behalf of the panel. The committee's main role is to advise the panel on procedural coding and nomenclature relevant to each member's specialty. The committee also provides documentation on medical and surgical procedures and suggests revisions to CPT.

Requests for Updating CPT

The process by which changes to the coding system are accomplished is described by the AMA as "deliberate." A specific pathway is followed when suggestions are received for revision of CPT. The steps in the process are as follows (American Medical Association 1992a):

1. AMA staff of physicians and coding experts evaluate all coding suggestions.
2. If the inquiry has been recently addressed by the CPT Editorial Panel, the requester is informed of the panel's interpretation.
3. If the request is a new issue, or if significant new information is received on an item that has been previously reviewed by the panel, the request is referred to the

appropriate members of the CPT Advisory Committee. In most cases, CPT Advisory Committee members have a formal network of advisers from within their own subspecialty and generally serve as chairpersons of that subspecialty's coding, reimbursement, or medical service committee. (The APA's network of advisers form the APA Work Group on Codes and Reimbursements, with the chairperson of the Work Group serving as the APA's representative to the CPT Advisory Committee.)

4. If the advisers that have been contacted agree that no new code or revision is needed, then AMA staff respond to the request with information on how existing codes should be used to report the procedure.

5. If the contacted advisers concur that a change should be made, or if two or more advisers disagree or give conflicting information, the issue is then referred to the CPT Editorial Panel for resolution. In making its decisions, the panel will ask the following questions:

    a. Is this a service that a physician may perform or a hospital-provided service mandated to be reported to a payer?

    b. Has the procedure/service been generally accepted by the medical community as evidenced by

    - Peer reviewed medical literature?
    - Assessment of a nationally recognized technology assessment agency program?
    - Specialty society evaluation?
    - Other available information?

    c. Is this procedure/service in widespread use? If not, does it represent a significant advance in medical practice? If so, is it advanced beyond research/investigation?

- Data from medical literature and, as available, from third-party payers concerning the frequency of use of the service or procedure will be reviewed as applicable.

d. Is this procedure/service adequately described by an existing code?

- Can an existing code be revised?
- Can modifiers be used with an existing code?

e. Does the procedure/service represent a different method of performing a given procedure or service? Does the technique substantially alter the management or outcome of a problem or condition and warrant a separate code?

The CPT Editorial Panel meets quarterly and relies on evidence of procedural safety and effectiveness as presented by the requester and specialty society advisers in making its decisions. There is one very important caveat—inclusion or exclusion of a procedure in CPT does not guarantee reimbursement.

The Medicare physician reimbursement system, the Resource-Based Relative Value Scale (RBRVS), has caused the addition of a step in the process of editing CPT. In collaboration with HCFA, the AMA has established a new committee—the RVS Update Committee (RUC)—whose purpose is to develop relative values for new or revised procedures. The RUC is composed of physician representatives from 22 specialty societies in addition to a representative from the AMA, who serves as the chairperson of the RUC and a member of the CPT Editorial Panel. The committee was established in November 1991.

Organization of *Physicians' Current Procedural Terminology, 4th Edition*

Introduction

The introduction to the fourth edition of CPT contains many important instructions about the manual. You must read this section to maximize your use of the manual. The introduction includes basic ground rules for using CPT, a description of its format, instructions for requesting updates for CPT, instructions on using modifiers, guidelines for coding unlisted procedures or services, and suggestions on special reports. The introduction also provides information about versions of CPT recorded on various formats (including computer tapes and diskettes), along with technical descriptions of the tapes and suggestions about compatible software.

Evaluation and Management Services

See the discussion on this section in Chapter 4.

Sections on Anesthesia, Surgery, Radiology, Pathology and Laboratory, and Medicine

The next five sections describe codes and procedures for specific medical services. Medicine is the last section of the manual, following Pathology and Laboratory. The Medicine section includes the codes for psychiatric evaluation and therapeutic procedures and begins with guidelines and a description of modifiers for use with the section. You should read these instructions carefully in order to fully understand the use of modifiers with psychiatric codes. The codes and modifiers will be reviewed in detail in Chapter 3.

Appendix A

Appendix A contains a complete list of all the modifiers in CPT. Modifiers that apply to each section are listed in the guidelines that begin the section.

Appendix B

Appendix B is a summary of the additions, deletions, and revisions to codes made in the current year. The codes are listed in numerical order with a notation next to each code indicating whether the code is new, has been changed, or has been deleted. When a code has been deleted from CPT, a reference will be made to a code to be used in place of the deleted code.

Appendix C

CPT comes not only in a book form but also is available on two tapes—one full and one short—and a diskette. The full tape contains the complete procedural text of the CPT manual, constructed in an 80-byte-per-line record. The short descriptive tape and the floppy disk contain the complete listing of codes found in CPT, but each has an abbreviated narrative written in nontechnical terms, with the code and the description limited to 28 characters or less on a single line. Appendix C contains all of the revisions from the prior year for the short procedure tape.

Appendix D

Appendix D is a clinical examples supplement. This new appendix contains clinical examples illustrating the use of CPT codes in various clinical settings.

Index

The Index of CPT is an alphabetical listing of main terms and consists of four primary classes of entries: 1) procedure or service (e.g., *Psychiatric Diagnosis* [the principal form of entry for psychiatric diagnostic services or procedures]); 2) organ or anatomic site (e.g., *brain*); 3) condition (e.g., *meningioma*); and 4) synonyms, eponyms, and abbreviations (e.g., *EEG, CAT scan, Dandy operation*). The instructions for using the index also describe modifying terms, code ranges, cross-references, and a number of other conventions. To use the index fully, it is important that you use these instructions.

Psychiatry Subsection

The Psychiatry subsection (American Medical Association 1997, pp. 351–354) is organized by the following headings: "Psychiatric Diagnostic or Evaluative Interview Procedures" and "Psychiatric Therapeutic Procedures." The latter heading is divided into "Office or Other Outpatient Facility"; "Inpatient Hospital, Partial Hospital, or Residential Care Facility"; "Other Psychotherapy"; and "Other Psychiatric Services or Procedures." Each procedure includes a description of the procedure. However, some procedures are not given a full descriptor but refer to a common portion of the descriptor for the preceding procedure, for example:

90804   Individual psychotherapy, insight oriented, behavior modifying, and/or supportive, in an office or outpatient facility, approximately 20–30 minutes face-to-face with the patient.

90805   with medical evaluation and management services.

Code Changes

Deleted Codes

When codes are deleted from CPT, a parenthetical notation is placed where the code had been located. The note will indicate that the code has been deleted and will refer to another code to use in its place, as the following example shows:

      (**90830** has been deleted. To report, use **96100**.)

Changes

A black circle (●) is placed before new procedure numbers added to CPT. A black triangle (▲) is placed before codes that have been revised by substantial alterations of the procedure descriptor. Triangular brackets (▶ ◀) indicate new or revised text.

Notations

Under the Psychiatry subsection in the Medicine section are a series of notes that provide guidance on selecting and using the psychiatric codes. These are very important instructions and should be read carefully. For example, the first notation guides the coder to the evaluation and management codes for psychiatric inpatient or partial hospitalization services. The notation describes the responsibilities unique to the medical management of psychiatric inpatients and lists the services attending physicians provide to patients on inpatient units. Another notation suggests which modifiers to use for unusual appointment lengths of individual medical psychotherapy. These notations are very helpful for coding usual procedures or procedures that are modified. The notations for special clinical psychiatric diagnostic or evaluative procedures describe the new interactive codes and are very helpful for understanding the use of these codes.

Questions and Answers

1. **How do I make suggestions about the introduction of new, or modifications of existing, procedures in CPT?**
   Send your suggestions to the Office of Economic Affairs and Practice Management, American Psychiatric Association, 1400 K Street, N.W., Washington, DC 20005, or the Department of Coding and Nomenclature, American Medical Association, 515 North State Street, Chicago, IL 60610.

2. **Do I really need to have an updated version of CPT every year?**

   Yes, because there are additions and modifications every year. For example, the individual psychotherapy codes have undergone a major revision in CPT 98.

3. **Why don't insurance companies pay for all the procedures listed in CPT?**

   CPT is a coding system only. Insurance companies voluntarily use the system but are not legally bound to pay for any procedure listed in the coding system.

4. **Are there any sections of the manual other than the section for psychiatry that are relevant to my practice as a psychiatrist?**

   As a physician, you are entitled to use any of the codes in the manual. You should have particular interest in the Evaluation and Management section because there are codes for many services that you most likely perform for your patients.

CHAPTER 3

Codes for Psychiatric Services

In this chapter, the codes most frequently used by psychiatrists are described. Many of the codes are in the Psychiatry subsection of the Medicine section (American Medical Association 1997, pp. 351–354). The introductory notes on psychiatry and the notes on each of its subsections provide guidance on how to select and use the codes. For example, the notations for psychiatry tell the clinician when to use the evaluation and management (E/M) codes **99221–99223** to code services provided by the attending physician for the first day of treatment of inpatients or partial hospitalization patients. When psychiatrists provide both E/M services and other procedures, such as electroconvulsive therapy or medical psychotherapy, the notes recommend that these services be listed separately. The notes instruct the physician to use a modifier (-52) to signify a service that is reduced or less extensive than usual and a modifier (-22) to indicate a service that is more extensive than usual.

The headings in the subsection on psychiatry are as follows:

- Psychiatric Diagnostic or Evaluative Interview Procedures
- Psychiatric Therapeutic Procedures

Psychiatric Diagnostic or Evaluative Interview Procedures

90801 Psychiatric diagnostic interview examination

This is *the* code most psychiatrists would use for the initial psychiatric evaluation of a new adult or adolescent patient. The diagnostic interview includes a chief complaint, history of present illness, review of systems, family and psychosocial history, and complete mental status examination, as well as the ordering and medical interpretation of laboratory or other medical diagnostic studies. This procedure is covered by all insurance carriers. Most carriers will reimburse the practitioner one time per patient per episode of illness. Medicare will pay for only one evaluation per year for institutionalized (i.e., nursing home) patients unless medical necessity for additional evaluations can be documented. According to Medicare payment policies, the psychiatrist may use this code or the appropriate level of the E/M codes

(**99221–99223**) to denote the initial evaluation or first-day services for hospitalized patients.

90802   Interactive psychiatric diagnostic interview examination using play equipment, physical devices, language interpreter, or other mechanisms of communication

In using this code, the psychiatrist is required to use physical aids or nonverbal communication to overcome barriers to therapeutic interaction between the psychiatrist and a patient who has impaired communication skills or who has not yet developed expressive language communication skills. This code was designed to be used primarily for the evaluation of young children but also may be used for adults who have impaired cognitive abilities. This is a covered service by all insurance plans, but medical necessity for use of the code must be documented. Several psychiatrists have been found guilty of fraudulent billing because of regular use of this code with adult patients for whom medical necessity could not be demonstrated.

Psychiatric Therapeutic Procedures

In CPT '98, the subsection on psychiatric therapeutic procedures has undergone major changes. The text provides a general definition of psychotherapy and indicates the codes are divided into two categories: 1) interactive psychotherapy and 2) insight-oriented, behavior-modifying, and/or supportive psychotherapy. The two categories of therapy are defined and are of utmost importance. Psychotherapy is *unbundled* from continuing medical diagnostic evaluation and drug management. Psychotherapy may now be provided and coded *with* and *without* medical E/M services. Psychotherapy with E/M services (medical diagnostic E/M services) will be reimbursed at a higher rate than psychotherapy without E/M services (pure psychotherapy) because the total work (intraservice and pre-/postservice) of psychotherapy with E/M is greater. The text also indicates the site of service should differentiate between office and inpatient settings (inpatient psychotherapy will be reimbursed at a higher rate). Thus, the appropriate code is selected based on

- Face-to-face time spent with the patient during psychotherapy
- Interactive psychotherapy versus insight-oriented, behavior-modifying, or supportive psychotherapy
- With E/M services versus without E/M services
- Outpatient/office versus inpatient

The text instructs, "to report medical evaluation and management services furnished on a day when psychotherapy is not provided, select the appropriate code from the Evaluation and Management Services Guidelines."

Individual psychotherapy as now defined by the category listed above results in 24 new codes organized in the following manner:

Office or Other Outpatient Facility

Insight-oriented, behavior-modifying, and/or supportive psychotherapy
- 90804   20–30 minutes
- 90805   20–30 minutes with E/M
- 90806   45–50 minutes
- 90807   45–50 minutes with E/M
- 90808   75–80 minutes
- 90809   75–80 minutes with E/M

Interactive psychotherapy
  - 90810   20–30 minutes
  - 90811   20–30 minutes with E/M
  - 90812   45–50 minutes
  - 90813   45–50 minutes with E/M
  - 90814   75–80 minutes
  - 90815   75–80 minutes with E/M

Inpatient Hospital, Partial Hospital, or Residential Care Facility

Insight-oriented, behavior-modifying, and/or supportive psychotherapy
  - 90816   20–30 minutes
  - 90817   20–30 minutes with E/M
  - 90818   45–50 minutes
  - 90819   45–50 minutes with E/M
  - 90821   75–80 minutes
  - 90822   75–80 minutes with E/M

Interactive psychotherapy
  - 90823   20–30 minutes
  - 90824   20–30 minutes with E/M
  - 90826   45–50 minutes
  - 90827   45–50 minutes with E/M
  - 90828   75–80 minutes
  - 90829   75–80 minutes with E/M

As you can see from the above lists, the codes for individual psychotherapy have been extensively revised. For a full understanding of these changes and any future modifications, you must obtain and read the annually published CPT.

Other Psychotherapy

90845   Psychoanalysis

Psychoanalysis is a form of psychotherapy that relies on elic-
iting from patients ideas of their past emotional experiences
and the facts of their mental life in order to discover the
mechanisms by which a pathologic mental state had been
produced and to furnish hints for psychotherapeutic procedures. Psychoanalysis is performed by therapists who are
trained and credentialed to practice psychoanalysis. The
procedure is reported on a per-session basis and is reimbursed by most insurance programs. The issue of medical
necessity has resulted in challenges to reimbursement for
this procedure by managed care companies.

90846 Family psychotherapy (without patient present)

The code is used when the psychiatrist provides therapy for
the family of the patient without the patient being present.
This code is reimbursed by most insurance companies; however, challenges to reimbursement may occur because the
service is not face-to-face with the patient.

90847 Family psychotherapy (conjoint psychotherapy)
            (with patient present)

This code is used when the therapy includes the patient and
family members. This is a covered service by most insurance plans and is challenged less often than the former code
because it involves a face-to-face service to the patient.

90849 Multiple-family group psychotherapy

This code is used when the psychiatrist provides psychotherapy to a group (more than one) of adult or adolescent
patients and their family members. The usual treatment
strategy is to modify family behavior and attitudes. This service is covered by most insurance plans.

90853 Group psychotherapy (other than of a multiple-family group)

This procedure relies on the use of interactions of group members to examine the pathology of each individual patient within the group. In addition, the dynamics of the entire group are noted and used to modify behaviors and attitudes of the patient members. The size of the group may vary depending on the therapeutic goals of the group and/or the type of therapeutic interactions used by the therapist. The code is used to report a per-session service for each patient group member. This procedure is covered by most insurance programs.

90857 Interactive group psychotherapy

The code for this procedure is used when practitioners provide psychotherapy using nonverbal communication and activities such as play therapy with young children in groups. These methods are necessary because of limited or underdeveloped communication skills of the patients. Similar procedures might be necessary for adult patients who have impaired communication skills. Psychiatrists should not use this code routinely for adults unless medical necessity can be documented. All insurance companies, including Medicare, have begun auditing psychiatrists who routinely use this procedure for adults.

Other Psychiatric Services or Procedures

90862 Pharmacologic management, including prescription, use, and review of medication with no more than minimal medical psychotherapy

The code for pharmacologic management is used when the patient is being treated with psychotropic medication. The interval history and mental status examination of the patient in each session are focused on response to the medication and a review of side effects. Any psychotherapy provided during these sessions would be supportive and brief. It is not necessary to write a prescription each time this procedure is coded, but the patient must be on a medication. Because use of this code has substantially increased, the Health Care Financing Administration and commercial carriers have been reviewing and auditing use of the code. The code is covered by all insurance companies, but frequency of use of the code for a given patient must be based upon medical necessity with appropriate documentation.

90865 Narcosynthesis for psychiatric diagnostic and therapeutic purposes (e.g., sodium amobarbital [Amytal] interview)

This procedure involves the administration, usually through slow intravenous infusion, of a barbiturate or a benzodiazepine in order to suppress inhibitions, thus allowing the patient to reveal and discuss material that he or she is unable to verbalize without the disinhibiting effect of the medication. This code is reimbursed by most insurance programs.

90870 Electroconvulsive therapy (includes necessary monitoring); single seizure

90871   multiple seizures, per day

These codes are for electroconvulsive therapy. Electroconvulsive therapy involves the application of electric current to the patient's brain for the purposes of producing a convulsion or series of convulsions to alleviate mental symptoms. The procedure is used primarily for the treatment of depression. The codes include the time the physician takes in monitoring the patient during the convulsive phase itself and during the recovery phase. When the psychiatrist also administers the anesthesia for electroconvulsive therapy, the anesthesia service should be reported separately. The service is covered by all insurance plans.

90875 Individual psychophysiological therapy incorporating biofeedback training by any modality (face-to-face with the patient), with psychotherapy (e.g., insight oriented, behavior modifying, or supportive psychotherapy); approximately 20–30 minutes

90876 approximately 45–50 minutes

These two procedures incorporate biofeedback and psychotherapy (insight oriented, behavior modifying, or supportive) as combined modalities conducted face-to-face with the patient. They are distinct from biofeedback codes **90901** and **90911**, which do not incorporate psychotherapy and do not require face-to-face time. The codes are reimbursed by most insurers.

90880 Hypnotherapy

Hypnosis is the procedure of inducing a passive state in which the patient demonstrates increased amenability and responsiveness to suggestions and commands, provided they do not conflict seriously with the patient's conscious or unconscious wishes. Hypnotherapy may be used for either diagnostic or treatment purposes. This procedure is covered by most insurance plans.

90882 Environmental intervention for medical management purposes on a psychiatric patient's behalf with agencies, employers, or institutions

Activities reported under this code include physician visits to a work site to improve work conditions for a particular patient, visits to community-based organizations on behalf of a chronically mentally ill patient to discuss a change in living conditions, or accompaniment of a patient with a phobia in order to help desensitize the patient to a stimulus. Other activities include coordination of services with agencies, employers, or institutions. This service is covered by most insurance plans, but because some activities are not face-to-face, the clinician should check with carriers for their willingness to cover the service.

90885 Psychiatric evaluation of hospital records, other psychiatric reports, psychometric and/or projective tests, and other accumulated data for medical diagnostic purposes

Theoretically, this code should be very useful in this new era of managed care. The totality of data to be reviewed for each patient is substantial as patients migrate from one health plan to the next. However, because reviewing data is not a face-to-face service with the patient, Medicare, and probably some commercial carriers, will not reimburse for this code. Medicare considers the review of data as part of the pre-/postwork associated with any face-to-face service.

90887 Interpretation or explanation of results of psychiatric, other medical examinations and procedures, or other accumulated data to family or other responsible persons, or advising them how to assist patient

This code is used when the psychiatrist explains the results of tests and/or examinations to the family of a patient or to other responsible persons. Medicare no longer reimburses for this service because it is not done face-to-face with the patient, and the clinician must verify coverage by other insurance companies to ensure reimbursement.

90889   Preparation of report of patient's psychiatric status, history, treatment, or progress (other than for legal or consultative purposes) for other physicians, agencies, or insurance carriers

This code is used for the preparation of a report about the patient to another physician, agency, or insurance carrier. The code should not be used for consultations or for legal purposes. In today's medical practice environment, psychiatrists are called upon to prepare reports about the patient for many participants in the health care system. This code would be best used to denote those services. Because these services are not provided face-to-face with a patient, the psychiatrist should check with local carriers and commercial insurers regarding reimbursement for these services.

90899   Unlisted psychiatric service or procedure

This code would be used for services not specifically defined under another code. The code also might be used for procedures that require some degree of explanation or justification for a service. If the code is used under these circumstances, a brief, jargon-free note explaining the use of the code to the insurance carrier might be helpful in obtaining reimbursement for the service. If the service is not provided face-to-face with a patient, the psychiatrist should check with the Medicare carrier or the commercial insurance companies regarding reimbursement.

Central Nervous System Assessments/Tests (e.g., Neurocognitive, Mental Status, Speech Testing)

96100   Psychological testing (includes psychodiagnostic assessment of personality, psychopathology, emotionality, intellectual abilities, e.g., WAIS-R, Rorschach, MMPI) with interpretation and report, per hour

Testing reported under this code includes psychodiagnostic assessments of personality, psychopathology, emotionality, and intellectual abilities. The tests commonly used are the Wechsler Adult Intelligence Scale—Revised (WAIS-R), Rorschach, and Minnesota Multiphasic Personality Inventory. The total work effort includes interpretation and report and is coded per hour of work. The code is located in the section on central nervous system assessments/tests (American Medical Association 1997, p. 377). Most insurance plans cover these services; many plans will only reimburse psychologists for these services.

Assessment of higher cerebral function (or aphasia testing) with medical interpretation is reported with code **96105**. There are also codes for developmental testing (**96110**) and extended testing of development (**96111**). The code for neurobehavioral status examination is **96115**. The code for neuropsychological test battery, which includes Halstead-Reitan, Luria, and WAIS-R, is **96117**. These codes differentiate between the groups of tests that might be used to examine various patient capabilities. Each of the codes is specific for the set of tested functions, and insurers cover the testing services.

Evaluation and Management

The E/M codes are described in detail in Chapter 4.

Special Services and Reports

This subheading includes a series of codes for reporting the completion of special reports and services that are adjuncts to basic services to patients.

Miscellaneous Services

Handling and/or conveyance of specimens for transfer from the physician's office to a laboratory is reported with code **99000**. Handling and/or conveyance of specimens for transfer from the patient in other than a physician's office to a laboratory (distance may be indicated) is reported with code **99001**. Handling, conveyance, and/or any other service in connection with the implementation of an order involving devices (e.g., designing, fitting, packaging, handling, delivering, or mailing) when devices such as orthotics, protectives, and prosthetics are fabricated by an outside laboratory or shop but are designed, fitted, and adjusted by the attending physician is reported with code **99002**.

These codes are used to report the physician's time in handling specimens such as blood samples for diagnostic purposes. A physician also would use code **99002** for reporting light therapy and for instructing the patient in the setup of the equipment.

Services requested after office hours in addition to basic service are reported with code **99050**. Services requested between 10 P.M. and 8 A.M. in addition to basic service are reported with code **99052**. Services requested on Sundays and holidays in addition to basic service are reported with code **99054**. Services provided at the request of a patient in a location other than the physician's office, which are normally provided in the office, are reported with code **99056**. Office services provided on an emergency basis are reported with code **99058**.

Physicians use these codes for reporting services when there are unusual circumstances. A brief, jargon-free note explaining the necessity of using these codes for the services may be helpful in obtaining the appropriate reimbursement from the insurance carrier.

Supplies and materials (except spectacles) provided by

the physician over and above those usually included with the office visit or other services rendered (list drugs, trays, supplies, or materials provided) are reported with code **99070**. Educational supplies, such as books, tapes, and pamphlets, provided at cost to the physician for the patient's education are reported with code **99071**.

Physicians use these codes to report materials supplied to the patient for actual treatment and/or for improving the patient's compliance with treatment.

Code **99075**, medical testimony, is used by physicians to report time spent in providing depositions or court testimony pursuant to explaining the patient's medical status or in providing expert testimony.

Completing special reports such as insurance forms or reviewing medical data to clarify a patient's status—beyond the information conveyed in the usual medical communications or standard reporting forms—is reported with code **99080**. In today's practice climate, this code may be particularly useful for reporting the time spent completing complicated insurance forms or requests for information about the patient to justify treatment.

Code **99082** is used to report unusual travel by a physician who accompanies a patient requiring an escort from one location to another, including travel between cities or across continents.

The practitioner should check with the third-party carrier or commercial insurers for their payment policies regarding reimbursement for the previously described codes.

Modifiers

Modifiers are two-digit numbers added to procedural codes (e.g., **90807-22**) that indicate the procedure has been provided to the patient under special circumstances that do not alter the basic definition of the procedure. Without modifiers, many more procedural listings would be needed to represent a variety of circumstances. Modifiers are listed in the guidelines for each section and in Appendix A of the CPT manual. When reporting modified procedures to insurance carriers, you must remember to explain to the carrier the special circumstances that necessitated the use of the modifier to improve your chances of being reimbursed. The explanation should be a short note describing, in a factual, jargon-free manner, 1) the patient's problem, 2) the treatment provided, 3) the time and effort, and 4) the medical necessity of the altered procedure. The following is an example of an explanatory note for the use of a modifier:

> Extended Psychotherapy Session—**90807-22**
> **(65 minutes)**
>
> (Patient's name)
> (ID number)
> (Group number)
> (Date of service)
> (Your name and address)
>
> Dear _____:
>
> Mr. X was scheduled for a 50-minute psychotherapy session for the treatment of his depressive illness. Near the close of the session, he told me about the sudden onset of suicidal thoughts. These thoughts were of sufficient intensity to require an additional 15 minutes of work with Mr. X to review the symptoms and convince him of the necessity of hospitalization. The total time of the individual psychotherapy was 65 minutes.

Most of the modifiers used by psychiatrists are found in the guidelines of the Medicine section (American Medical

Association 1997, pp. 346–348). The following modifiers are most commonly used by psychiatrists:

-21 Prolonged evaluation and management services

This modifier is to be used when the work associated with the service provided is greater than that usually required for the highest level of an E/M service within a given category (see p. 387 of CPT).

-22 Unusual procedural services

This modifier is to be used when the work associated with the service provided is greater than that usually required for the listed procedure.

-26 Professional component

When procedures include a physician component and a technical component, the physician component can be reported separately by using this modifier.

-32 Mandated services

This modifier is used to report mandated consultations or services. An example of a mandated consultation is a second opinion for using electroconvulsive therapy. The confirmatory consultation codes **99271–99275** would be used with the addition of this modifier.

-52 Reduced services

This modifier is used to report a procedure that is reduced in work or time.

One important reminder: when reporting modified codes, include a brief explanatory note, an example of which has been shown earlier in this section.

Unlisted Service or Procedure

For reporting a service or procedure that is not listed in CPT, the code for psychiatry is **90899**. Practitioners reporting this code should include a short explanatory note similar to the one shown earlier as an example for reporting modifiers.

Questions and Answers

1. **What codes are most appropriate for reporting hospital care provided by an attending psychiatrist?**

   The notations for the Psychiatry subsection recommend using **99221–99233** (E/M hospital inpatient services). These codes most accurately reflect the diverse services provided by attending psychiatrists. For the initial day of care there may be an option (depending on the reimbursement policy of the involved insurance company) of using the E/M initial hospital care (**99221–99223**) or the psychiatric diagnostic interview code (**90801**). Codes for individual psychotherapy (inpatient hospital [**90816–90822**]) require the clinician to provide face-to-face psychotherapy to the patient each day the code is used. An attending physician who provides E/M hospital inpatient services and inpatient hospital individual psychotherapy on the same day may choose to code and bill for both services or code and bill for individual psychotherapy with medical E/M services. Medicare will pay for only one service per day for the attending physician. When attending physicians provide psychotherapy and E/M services on the same day to Medicare patients, they will most likely use **90817** (20–30 minutes), **90819** (45–50 minutes), or **90822** (75–80 minutes) because these codes have higher Relative Value Units and are better reimbursed than the E/M subsequent hospital care codes. But remember, you must provide face-to-face psychotherapy for the entire time coded. The E/M services are considered pre- or postprocedure (psychotherapy) work.

2. **Do all payers accept these psychiatric service codes?**
   Most payers accept these psychiatric service codes. However, Medicare only will reimburse providers for services that are provided face-to-face with the patient.

3. **Where are the codes for psychiatric services provided in partial hospital, residential treatment, and nursing homes located in CPT?**
   The codes for partial hospital services are the same as those used for hospital inpatient services (**99221–99233**), and codes for residential treatment services are the same as those used for nursing facility services (**99301–99313**).

4. **When would I use the pharmacologic management code (90862) rather than one of the E/M outpatient codes?**
   Your decision should be based on which code most accurately reports the services rendered. Code **90862** does not include levels representing increasing work effort; therefore, it does not require selecting one of the various levels of care (see Chapter 4).

5. **What code should I use for reporting psychotherapy provided by telephone?**
   There are two methods of reporting psychotherapy provided by telephone: 1) telephone calls (**99371–99373**) with an explanatory note or 2) unlisted procedure (**90899**) with an explanatory note. Choosing a method of reporting this service should be by agreement with

the payer before you start billing for occasional or routine provision of this service.

6. **If I provide a unique service on a recurrent basis, do I have to use a modifier and provide an explanatory note each time I report the service?**
Before reporting such services, you should reach an agreement with the carrier about 1) the payer's willingness to reimburse you for the service and 2) the payer's preferred method of reporting the service.

CHAPTER 4

Evaluation and Management Services

T he evaluation and management (E/M) codes were introduced in the fourth edition of *Physicians' Current Procedural Terminology* (CPT; American Medical Association 1992b). In 1994 and 1997, Medicare published revised guidelines for E/M code selection and levels of service. These codes cover general medical services provided at a variety of sites (e.g., office, hospital, nursing home, domiciliary care, patient's home). The codes are generic in the sense that they may be used by all physicians—primary and specialty care physicians alike. The definition of key terms and the method for selecting a level of service are explained in the Evaluation and Management

Services Guidelines section of CPT (American Medical Association 1997, pp. 1–8). It is important that you read this section so that you understand the basic principles established by CPT for selecting procedural codes and for choosing the appropriate level of service.

E/M codes include the following services:

- Office or other outpatient services
- Hospital observation services
- Hospital inpatient services
- Consultations
- Emergency department services
- Critical care services
- Neonatal intensive care services
- Nursing facility services
- Domiciliary, rest home, or custodial care services
- Home services
- Prolonged services
- Standby services
- Case management services
- Care plan oversight services
- Preventive medicine services
- Special E/M services
- Other E/M services

The format of the E/M section consists of broad categories of service with definitions of the services and specific directions for selecting codes within the category. The notations are very useful in helping you code accurately. The categories of service are generally divided into subcategories of new patient and established patient, and there are generally three or five levels of service. The format for each code is similar: [a]the number, [b]the place of service or type of service, [c]the content of the service, [d]the nature of the presenting problem(s) usually associated with a given level, and [e]the average time of service. Each of these components (see corresponding letter) is shown in the following example:

> [a]99254 [b]Initial inpatient consultation for a new or established patient, which requires three key components:
>
> - [c]a comprehensive history
> - [c]a comprehensive examination
> - [c]medical decision making of moderate complexity
>
> [d]Usually, the presenting problem(s) are of moderate to high severity. [e]Physicians typically spend 80 minutes at the bedside and on the patient's hospital floor or unit.

The definitions of new patient and established patient are important because of the extensive use of these terms throughout the guidelines in the E/M section. A *new patient* is defined as one who has not received any professional services from the physician or another physician of the same specialty who belongs to the same group within the past 3 years. An *established patient* is one who has received professional services from the physician or another physician of the same specialty who belongs to the same group within the past 3 years. When a physician is on call covering for another physician, the decision as to whether the patient is new or established is determined by the relationship of the physician to the patient for whom the coverage is being provided. There is no distinction made between new and established patients in the emergency department.

Level of Evaluation and Management Services

Each E/M service generally has three to five levels of service, based on the complexity of the case and the amount of attending work. The level of service is specific for each category of E/M service. Physician work includes history taking, physical and mental status examinations, treatments, patient and family conferences, ordering tests, and analyzing test results—in fact, all manner of medical services. Each level of service consists of several components:

- History
- Examination
- Medical decision making
- Counseling
- Coordination of care
- Nature of presenting problem
- Time

History, examination, and medical decision making are the key components for the selection of level of the E/M services. Counseling, coordination of care, and the nature of the presenting problem are contributory factors. Time is discussed in detail later in this section.

History

There are four levels of work associated with history taking:

1. *Problem focused:* chief complaint—brief history of present illness or problem
2. *Expanded problem focused:* chief complaint—brief history of present illness; problem-pertinent system review
3. *Detailed:* chief complaint—extended history of present illness; extended system review; pertinent past, family, and/or social history
4. *Comprehensive:* chief complaint—extended history of present illness; complete system review; complete past, family, and social history

Examination

There are four levels of work associated with performing a physical examination:

1. *Problem focused:* examination limited to affected body area or organ system
2. *Expanded problem focused:* examination of affected body area or organ system and other symptomatic or related organ systems
3. *Detailed:* extended examination of the affected body area(s) and other symptomatic or related organ system(s)
4. *Comprehensive:* complete single-system specialty examination or a complete multisystem examination (see Chapter 7)

Medical Decision Making

Medical decision making refers to the complex tasks of establishing a diagnosis and selecting a management option. There are three criteria resulting in four types of medical decision making.

Criteria:

1. Number of possible diagnoses and/or number of management options
2. Amount and/or complexity of medical records, diagnostic tests, and/or other information that must be obtained, reviewed, and analyzed
3. The risk of significant complications, morbidity, and/or mortality, as well as comorbidities associated with the patient's presenting problem(s), the diagnostic procedure(s), and/or possible management options

Types of medical decision making:

1. Straightforward
2. Low complexity
3. Moderate complexity
4. High complexity

   The factors leading to the different levels of medical decision making are shown in Table 4–1.

Counseling

Counseling is a discussion with a patient or a family concerning one or more of the following issues:

- Diagnostic results, impressions, and/or recommended diagnostic studies
- Prognosis
- Risks and benefits of management (treatment) options

Table 4–1. Criteria leading to level of medical decision making

Number of diagnoses or management options	Amount/ complexity of medical records	Risk	Medical decision[a]
Minimal	Minimal or none	Minimal	Straight-forward
Limited	Limited	Low	Low complexity
Multiple	Moderate	Moderate	Moderate complexity
Extensive	Extensive	High	High complexity

[a]When two of three criteria on same line have been met.

- Instructions for management (treatment) and/or follow-up
- Importance of compliance with chosen management (treatment) options
- Risk factor reduction
- Patient and family education

Coordination of Care

Coordination of care is not specifically defined in the Guidelines section, but a working definition of the term could be the following: services provided by the physician responsible for the direct care of a patient when he or she coordinates or controls access to care or initiates or supervises other health care services needed by the patient. Outpatient coordination of care must be provided face-to-face with the patient. Coordination of care with other providers or agencies without the patient being present on that day is reported using the case management codes.

Nature of Presenting Problem

A presenting problem is a disease, condition, illness, injury, symptom, sign, finding, complaint, or other reason for the encounter with the physician, with or without a diagnosis having been made. There are five categories of presenting problems:

1. *Minimal:* may not require the presence of a physician, but care is provided under physician's supervision
2. *Self-limited or minor:* problem runs a prescribed course, is transient in nature, is not likely to alter the health status permanently, or is one that has a good prognosis
3. *Low severity:* problem for which there is low risk of morbidity without treatment, low or no risk of mortal-

ity without treatment, or full recovery without functional impairment

4. *Moderate severity:* problem for which there is moderate risk of morbidity without treatment, moderate risk of mortality without treatment, and uncertain prognosis or increased probability of prolonged functional impairment

5. *High severity:* problem for which there is high to extreme risk of morbidity without treatment, moderate to high risk of mortality without treatment, or high probability of severe and prolonged functional impairment

Time

For the purpose of selecting the level of service, time has two definitions. You must review the E/M Guidelines section (American Medical Association 1997, p. 4) to understand completely the rationale for the two definitions.

For office and other outpatient visits and office consultations, intraservice time (time spent by the clinician providing services with the patient and/or family present) is defined as *face-to-face*. Pre- and postencounter time (non–face-to-face services) is not included in the average times listed under each level of service in office and outpatient consultative services. The work associated with pre- and postencounter time has been included in the total work effort provided by the physician for that service.

Time spent providing hospital observation services, inpatient hopsital care, initial and follow-up hospital consultations, and nursing facility services is defined as *unit/floor time*. Unit/floor time includes all the work the psychiatrist performs on behalf of the patient while present on the unit or at the bedside. Included in the unit/floor time is direct patient contact, reviewing charts, writing orders, reviewing test results, writing progress notes, meeting with the treatment team, handling telephone calls, and meeting with the patient's family. Pre- and posttime work, such as reviewing X rays in another part of the hospital, has been included in the calculation of the total work provided by the physician for that service.

The Guidelines section instructs you to use the three components for selecting the level of service except when counseling and/or coordination of care accounts for more than 50% of the patient and/or family encounter. In that instance, time becomes the key component for selecting the level of service whether it is an outpatient (face-to-face), hospital inpatient, or nursing facility service (unit/floor time). You select the level of service by matching the total time of the encounter to the average times listed for each level of service for the appropriate E/M service. For example, if you provide subsequent hospital care as an attending physician and counseling and coordination of care (e.g., meeting with the treatment team, making telephone calls to arrange aftercare, writing orders, reviewing test results) and these services constitute more than 50% of the total unit/floor time, time becomes the key component in selecting the level of service. The specific services provided under counseling and coordination of care must be documented in the medical record along with the time. Documentation issues are discussed in more detail in Chapter 7.

The relationship among the key component—time—and the components counseling and coordination of care is important. You spend a great deal of time with patients reviewing treatment plans, discussing the importance of compliance, talking with families, consulting with social agencies, participating in unit treatment team conferences, or completing commitment processes. All of this work can be captured under the definitions of time as described earlier. As a reminder, counseling and coordination of care in the office or in an outpatient setting must be provided face-to-face with the patient and/or the patient's family.

Selecting the Level of
Evaluation and Management Services

There are seven steps for selecting the appropriate level of an E/M service:

Step 1.   Select the category and subcategory of E/M service.   Table 4–2 lists the E/M services most likely to be used by psychiatrists. Keep in mind that Table 4-2 is only a partial list of codes; you will need to refer to CPT for the full listing of CPT codes.

Step 2.   Review the descriptors and reporting instructions for the E/M service selected.   Most of the categories and many of the subcategories have special guidelines or instructions governing the use of that E/M code. For example, under the description of initial hospital care for a new or established patient, the manual indicates that the inpatient care level of service reported by the admitting physician should include the services related to the admission that he or she provided in other sites of service, as well as in the inpatient setting. E/M services on the same date provided in sites other than the hospital that are related to the admission should *not* be reported separately (American Medical Association 1997, p. 15).

Step 3.   Review the service descriptors and the requirements for the key components for the selected E/M service.   Each category or subcategory of E/M service lists in boldface type the required level of history, examination, or medical decision making required for that particular code. Exceptions include the descriptor requirements for critical care services, case management services, preventive medicine services, and counseling or risk factor reduction intervention.

Table 4–2. Evaluation and management services most likely to be used by psychiatrists

Category/subcategory	Code numbers	CPT 98 page reference
Office or outpatient services		
New patient	99201–99205	pp. 9–11
Established patient	99211–99215	pp. 11–13
Hospital inpatient services		
Initial hospital care	99221–99223	pp. 15–16
Subsequent hospital care	99231–99233	pp. 17–18
Hospital discharge services	99238	p.19
Consultations		
Office consultations	99241–99245	pp. 20–22
Initial inpatient consultations	99251–99255	pp. 22–24
Follow-up inpatient consultations	99261–99263	pp. 24–26
Confirmatory consultations	99271–99275	pp. 26–27
Emergency department services	99281–99288	pp. 27–29
Nursing facility services		
Comprehensive nursing facility assessments	99301–99303	pp. 31–33
Subsequent nursing facility care	99311–99313	pp. 33–34
Domiciliary, rest home, or custodial care services		
New patient	99321–99323	pp. 34–35

(continued)

Table 4–2.   Evaluation and management services most likely to be used by psychiatrists (*continued*)

Category/subcategory	Code numbers	CPT 98 page reference
Established patient	99331–99333	p. 35
Home services		
New patient	99341–99343	pp. 35–36
Established patient	99351–99353	pp. 36–37
Case management services		
Team conferences	99361–99362	p. 39
Telephone calls	99371–99373	p. 39
Preventive medicine services		
New patient	99381–99387	p. 40
Established patient	99391–99397	p. 41
Individual counseling	99401–99404	p. 41
Group counseling	99411–99412	p. 41
Other	99420–99429	p. 41
Other evaluation and management services	99499	p. 42

Note. Page numbers refer to the 1998 *Physicians' Current Procedural Terminology* (CPT). CPT codes and descriptions are © 1997 American Medical Association. All Rights Reserved.

Step 4.   Determine the extent of work required in obtaining the history.   The four levels of history have been described previously in this chapter under the History section.

Step 5.   Determine the extent of work performed in obtaining the examination.   The four levels of examination have been described previously in this chapter under the Examination section.

Step 6. Determine the complexity of medical decision making. The grid for selecting the level of medical decision making is shown in Table 4–1.

Step 7. Select the appropriate level of E/M service.

1. For new patients, the three key components (history, examination, and medical decision making) must meet or exceed the stated requirements to qualify for each level of service for office visit, initial hospital care, office consultations, initial inpatient consultations, confirmatory consultations, emergency department services, comprehensive nursing facility assessments, domiciliary care, and home services.

2. For established patients, two of the three key components (history, examination, and medical decision making) must meet or exceed the stated requirements to qualify for each level of service for office visit, subsequent hospital care, follow-up inpatient consultations, subsequent nursing facility care, domiciliary care, and home care.

3. When counseling and coordination of care account for more than 50% of the face-to-face physician-patient encounter, then time becomes the key or controlling factor in selecting the level of service. Note that counseling or coordination of care must be documented in the medical record.

All of the E/M codes are available to you for reporting your services. The codes for hospital inpatient services; consultation services; emergency department services; nursing facility services; domiciliary, rest home, or custodial care services; home services; case management services; preventive medicine services; and counseling or risk factor reduction intervention are used by psychiatrists.

Many psychiatrists use hospital inpatient service and consultation codes frequently. Practitioners frequently ask, "Under what clinical circumstances would you use the office or other outpatient service codes in lieu of the psychiatric evaluation and psychiatric therapy codes?" The decision to use one set of codes versus another will be based on which code most accurately describes the services provided to the patient. The E/M codes give you flexibility for reporting your services. Please note that although there are now many codes available to use for reporting services, the existence of the codes in CPT does not guarantee reimbursement from any third-party payer. (Third-party relationships are discussed in Chapter 5.)

Questions and Answers

1. **May psychiatrists use E/M codes?**
    Yes. Attempts by certain carriers to restrict access are not consistent with CPT or federal policy. If you are denied use of E/M codes, contact your district branch and local medical society. Seek assistance through the medical director of the carrier.

2. **Is a unit treatment team conference on an inpatient unit a codable service?**
    Treatment team conferences should be considered coordination of care. The time spent providing that service is a component of the total unit/floor time. Team conferences should not be coded as a separate service but rather as a component of the total services provided to the patient on any given day.

3. **If I have a patient in the hospital whom I see for rounds in the morning and again when I am called to the ward in the afternoon because of a problem, do I**

code for two subsequent hospital care visits?

No. One code should be selected that incorporates all of the hospital inpatient services provided that day.

4. **How do I code for the time it takes me to complete commitment proceedings on a patient?**

You would have the option of using the psychiatric evaluation code **90801** and modifier **-22**, if the service required an unusual length of time, or an office service code at the appropriate level of service. If you select an office visit code, only the time spent face-to-face with the patient may be used to calculate the level of service. Should the face-to-face time associated with commitment proceedings be unusually lengthy, use the **-21** modifier. Attach a brief explanatory note to the billing form.

5. **What are the requirements associated with outpatient consultations?**

The request for the consultation must be documented in the patient's medical record. The consultant's opinion and any services that are performed also must be documented in the patient's medical record and communicated to the requesting physician.

6. **How many follow-up outpatient consultation visits can I code for? How many inpatient consultation visits?**

None. Follow-up visits in the consultant's office or other outpatient facility that are initiated by the physician consultant are reported using office visit codes for established patients.

Theoretically, there is no limit to the number of follow-up inpatient consultation visits for recommending management modifications, advising on a new treatment plan, or responding to changes in the patient's status. When the consultant takes over any aspect of the patient's care, codes that appropriately describe the services provided by the physician should be used rather than follow-up consultation codes. Some insurance plans may limit the number of follow-up visits for which you can be reimbursed.

CHAPTER 5

Health Insurance Issues

Role of Health Insurance Companies in the Medical System

Following World War II, insurance companies successfully developed and marketed health insurance to millions of Americans. Large employers were willing to give employees health benefits (which were relatively inexpensive) in lieu of salary increases. Health insurance policies were designed to help patients pay for the cost of routine care and protect them from the cost of extraordinary medical expenses. Individuals and families buy medical benefits—the services covered by the policies—for dollars paid to providers of medical services. In general, the more expensive the premium, the greater the number of health services covered by the policy.

Except for Kaiser on the West Coast and the Health Insurance Plan in New York City, most health insurance programs were developed as indemnity plans.

For 30 years, health insurance appeared to be a financially successful, publicly supported policy. Patients were satisfied, physicians and other providers were reimbursed on a usual and customary fee-for-service basis, and the insurance companies made money. During the 1960s, the federal government addressed the problems of insurance for the poor and aging by developing Medicaid and Medicare. By the early 1970s, most individuals were covered by either private, state-federal, or federal health insurance programs. The public had come to expect health insurance, much of it seemingly paid for by someone else (employer or government), as an essential component of the health system.

Changes in the Health System

During the past 15 years, the increasing cost of medical care has led to novel forms of health insurance, which in turn have radically altered the practice environment. Patients have been required to bear a greater share of the costs of their premiums because employers' costs for health care benefits have increased sharply and eroded their profits. Insurance companies have developed a bewildering array of products in addition to traditional indemnity plans (e.g., health maintenance organizations [HMOs], preferred provider organizations (PPOs), and point-of-service contracts) and also have developed a variety of cost management techniques (e.g., utilization review, preauthorization for services, concurrent review of services, retrospective review of services, second opinions for certain services, and carve-out programs for management of mental health services). Competition for patients has required physicians to participate in these new forms of health care, resulting in erosion of fee for service and an increase in deeply discounted fees associated with PPO and HMO capitated contracts. Finally, as if these changes were not enough, a physician's work life has become a nightmare of paperwork.

Health policy experts expound on the adversarial relationship among patients, doctors, and insurance companies and suggest that the health system in America is in the process of melting down. For at least 10 years, the public has been told by various government agencies that the escalation of health care costs is the fault of physicians because of inflated fees, high incomes, waste, and fraud.

The impact of changes in the practice environment is pervasive. Patients are upset with physicians' and health insurance companies' increased costs. Insurance companies complain about patients overusing services and accuse physicians of inflating charges. Physicians are wary of patients who demand quality care at discounted fees and are ready to pounce on any medical outcome that is less than perfect. The relationship between physicians and health insurance companies is strained because cost management techniques have intruded into physician decision making. Unfortunately, within the context of this environment, you must manage the business aspects of your practice.

Organization

Insurance companies are large organizations with many levels of management. Most companies employ physicians in a variety of positions, including medical director, and most companies have a medical advisory board composed of community physicians who serve voluntarily. Nonphysician medical representatives are usually employed to help service relationships with physician providers. Despite the layers of management, which include physicians and specific programs for provider relations, practitioners often have difficulty accessing the decision-making apparatus of health insurance organizations.

Claims Management and Review

One of the most important activities of the insurance companies is processing claims. You would expect this activity to be a high priority for insurance companies. However, claims processing causes more problems and frustration for patients, physicians, and the companies themselves than any other aspect of their business operations. Despite the fact that claims processing is central to the function of a health insurance company, it remains a relatively low-tech, trouble-plagued operation.

Claims processing begins in the mail room of the insurance company, where attachments to a claim are removed along with staples and paper clips in preparation for processing. The claim then goes to the claims processors, who are typically young, high-school graduates paid minimum wage. The processors usually are not trained in medical terminology or coding. The task of the processors is to sort the claims and enter them into their computer terminals or return the claims because they are incomplete. Claims returned include those with missing diagnoses, dates of service, or signatures. The claims processors are required to process a certain number of claims within a given time period, whether the claims are entered or returned. Claims returned for missing data take a fraction of the time required to enter processed claims. Therefore, when behind in their work, processors can meet their quotas by returning claims whether they are missing information or not. When pressed for time, processors return claims for more information because that task is easier than processing the claim. The potential pitfalls of claims processing are one good reason for submitting claims electronically rather than manually, because the claims processor is bypassed.

Once entered into the computer system, the claim is reviewed by a claims examiner, who also typically has a high-school education, is paid a relatively low wage, and has limited training in medical terminology and coding. If the examiner understands the claim and agrees with the medical necessity for the service or procedure, payment will be authorized. However, if the examiner does not understand what was done to the patient and why it was done, he or she may take one of three actions: 1) return the claim to you for more information, 2) refer the claim for review at a higher technical level (nurse or physician review), or 3) file the claim, which often leads to a delayed decision or disappearance of the claim.

Clearly, problems for your claim can occur anywhere within the process. Strategies to protect your claim are discussed in Chapter 8.

Oversight

Insurance companies are regulated in each state by the office of an insurance commissioner. The responsibility of the commissioner is to ensure companies comply with state laws, maintain sufficient reserves, and conduct yearly audits. In addition to the oversight provided by the commissioner, the public service role of insurance companies attracts the attention of state legislators. The companies in turn employ lobbyists to influence the development of legislation beneficial to their operations. For the most part, their lobbying efforts are effective and balance the controls of the state insurance commissioner.

The Ideal Relationship Among Company, Patient, and Physician

The relationship among the patient, the health insurance company, and the physician should be interdependent and collaborative. Patients buy health insurance policies, physicians provide health care, and insurance carriers process claims and reimburse providers. Naturally occurring tensions among the three parties may be associated with 1) cost of the insurance, an issue for patient and insurance company; 2) uninsured costs (e.g., copayments), an issue for the patient and insurance company and for the patient and physician; and 3) claims processing and speed of reimbursement, an issue for the patient, physician, and insurance company. Ideally, these tensions can be managed to each of the three parties' satisfaction. Many patients and physicians would argue that the ideal relationship among the three involved parties has never existed.

Strategies for Dealing With Third-Party Carriers

If you understand the goals of the carriers, their priorities, their function within the health system, and their organization, you are well on your way to developing effective strategies for dealing with them.

Developing and Maintaining Relationships With Insurance Companies

1. *Maintain businesslike, cordial relationships with the insurance company and its personnel.* No matter how frustrated you may become, always remember the company has many ways of retaliating. It can slow processing of your claims, slow reimbursement, and, most troublesome of all, audit you.
2. *Do not be intimidated by the insurance company.* Your relationship with the insurance company is strictly business, and there are rules and regulations that it must obey. The state insurance commissioner, the

Better Business Bureau, the local medical society, the local psychiatric society, and your legislators may be useful resources in selected incidents or disputes with a health insurance company (see When Things Go Wrong, later in this chapter).

3. *Remember that an insurance company's first priority is its customer—your patient.* Both you and the insurance company are providing a service to your patient. Within the boundaries of concerns about transference-countertransference issues, keep your patient informed about both good and bad aspects of your business relationship with the insurance company and health plan. The feedback you provide the patient may affect his or her own interactions with the company.

4. *Develop and maintain contact with one or two employees in each insurance company.* You or your office manager should foster friendly relationships with people in each insurance company with which you deal. If you succeed in developing such relationships, you will have people inside the companies who know you and can help solve problems.

5. *Consider filing a record of your mode of practice with the insurance company.* Many group practices place on record with carriers their mode of practice, including the services they intend to provide, any unusual features of their practice (e.g., group rather than solo coverage of inpatient services), the codes to be used for reporting, a list of the individual providers, and the fees they intend to charge. The benefits of placing this information on record with the carrier are 1) problems with the mode of practice can be identified in advance and dealt with prospectively, 2) the record is a baseline set of data that helps the company make adjustments when any aspect of practice is changed, 3) the recorded mode also may serve as protection when disputes are caused by

changes in company policies or operations not communicated to the provider, and 4) the record may serve as a protection when disputes trigger audits. The person to contact in the insurance company in order to record your mode of practice or changes in your mode is the medical director of the company. The second choice for contact is the medical policy division.

6. *Document all contacts with insurance companies.* Keep all written materials that pass between you and insurance companies on file. Whenever you contact a company by telephone, record the name of the person with whom you spoke, his or her telephone number, and the date of the contact. As a follow-up to the telephone contact, send a memo to that person with a short, clear synopsis of the content of the call. If certain verbal agreements were made, document those agreements.

7. *Stay informed about the insurance companies with whom you do business.* Most companies periodically publish newsletters or directives to providers; read them carefully. Local and national newspapers regularly carry stories about insurance companies; although they may make for dry reading, the stories could contain useful information. Other sources of information about insurance companies and their operations and products are the American Psychiatric Association's (APA's) *EcoFacts*, your local psychiatric society, and your local medical society.

When Things Go Wrong

The likelihood that you eventually will have a significant dispute with an insurance company is high. Because every claim represents a portion of your revenue stream, you must follow up assertively on all returned or rejected claims.

1. *Remember, when dealing with an insurance company, it is business—nothing personal.* You are dealing with a large, impersonal bureaucracy that has many resources and means of retaliation. Keep your contacts business-like and cordial.

2. *Be persistent in your efforts to resolve any disputes.* Only you can decide how much effort should be expended in resolving any given dispute. But remember that repeated, businesslike contacts will eventually gain you access to an individual who can make decisions and help you.

3. *Enlist the help of your patient.* Remember that your patient is the insurance company's customer and its first priority. If you are making no progress, ask the patient to inquire about the disputed claim(s). The patient's request may be addressed while yours continues to be shuffled about. A patient's request for review of a claim usually requires some paperwork. It is in your best interest to help the patient complete the required paperwork. Information about health plan benefits and the mechanics of resolving disputed claims also may be available from the employee's company benefits manager (usually in the human resources department).

4. *Determine if there are any mechanisms for appeal.* If you cannot resolve an issue, ask the insurance company or insurance plan for the details of the formal appeals process.

5. *Look for help.* The following are some options:
   a. *Peers.* Your colleagues are an important source of information about insurance problems. Describe your problem to several physician friends; they may have had similar problems, and their experiences may provide answers for you. If the problem is shared by other physicians, consider a presentation

to the insurance committee of your local psychiatric society.

b. *Local psychiatric society.*   Most local psychiatric societies have standing insurance committees or committees on third-party relationships. These committees act as a clearinghouse for members who have problems with insurance companies. The knowledge and experience of the committees are often helpful to members who have disputes with insurance carriers. (The local medical society also may be helpful.) If the local psychiatric society is unable to assist you, it can turn to the parent organization, the APA.

c. *American Psychiatric Association.*   The APA has many resources for addressing members' problems with insurance companies. Three committees are dedicated to important aspects of the business relationships between psychiatrists and third-party carriers: the Committee on Managed Care, the Work Group on the Harvard Resource-Based Relative Value Scale, and the Work Group on Codes and Reimbursements. The chairpersons and staff of the committees regularly respond to members' inquiries about insurance and coding issues. In addition, members can influence APA policy concerning third-party carriers through their representatives to the APA's Assembly of District Branches. The current working relationship between the Assembly and the APA Board of Trustees guarantees that leadership attends to the insurance problems experienced by members.

d. *Legal counsel.*   From time to time there will be disputes with insurance companies that require use of legal counsel. The cost of legal expertise is usually prohibitive for the practitioner, but if colleagues are experiencing the same problem, the shared cost may be affordable. The best way to determine the impact of your problem on your peers is through your local psychiatric society. The society may even organize and financially support a legal strategy to solve a problem.

e. *Insurance commissioner.* If you believe your problem with a company represents a significant breach of the regulations governing the operation of insurance companies in your state, you can request the commissioner's review. This review is serious business, and such requests should not be made in anger or frivolously.

Again, if you use any or all of these suggestions, remember that your dispute with a company is a business issue—no matter how that issue personally affects you. Be cordial but determined.

Questions and Answers

1. **How can I protect my claims from being returned to me for what seem to be minor reasons?**
   Fill out the forms completely and legibly. Stamp or write on attachments, "please do not separate attachments." (See also Chapter 8.)

2. **How can my local psychiatric society help me when I have problems with an insurance company?**
   Your local psychiatric society can help in several ways. It can

   • Put you in touch with colleagues who have similar problems
   • Work with the insurance company to resolve the problem on behalf of you and other members

- Assist you in accessing APA resources
- Sponsor legislation
- Organize and sponsor legal actions

3. **Is it ethical to tell patients about problems I am having with their insurance companies?**

   Informing patients about your problems with their insurance companies is not unethical. In fact, asking patients for their assistance in resolving a disputed claim by suggesting that they request a review of the claim is a helpful tactic.

4. **Can I realistically expect to challenge one of these big companies over any issue?**

   A single practitioner will have difficulty influencing a company. By joining together with colleagues and enlisting the aid of the local psychiatric society and/or APA (e.g., Managed Care Help Line, [800] 343-4671), you gain the strength of group action, which may succeed when your individual effort would not.

5. **How can HMOs or managed care companies restrict physician access to certain service codes?**

   The CPT manual and its codes are conventions for reporting and recording services. Therefore, insurance and managed care companies may specify which service codes physicians can and cannot use

CHAPTER 6

Medicare

The Medicare program was established in 1965 to provide medical health benefits to individuals older than age 65 and individuals younger than age 65 who are considered disabled according to various government programs. Payments for health services are provided by Part A (payments for hospital services) and Part B (payments for physician services). Over the years the program has grown to become one of the largest payers of health care in the United States. You may ask why it is relevant to know about the Medicare program when your practice has few if any Medicare patients. You need to be informed about the Medicare program because many elements of the program (including the Resource-Based Relative Value Scale [RBRVS] for physician reimbursement) are being adopted by many commercial carriers.

Basic Payment Mechanism

Physician services provided on a *fee-for-service* basis ("traditional Medicare") are paid as follows: Medicare patients must pay a $100 annual deductible for Part B services, after which they pay a copayment of 20% of the Medicare-allowed amount for all subsequent Part B services. For outpatient psychiatric services, Medicare reduces the allowed amount to 62.5% of the fee schedule amount. The copayment for outpatient psychotherapy services is 50% ($62.5\% \times 80\% = 50\%$). Physician services not covered by Medicare are not reimbursed by the program and are the patient's responsibility. Physicians have the option of participating in Medicare for reimbursement. When a physician participates and accepts assignment, the patient's out-of-pocket financial responsibility is limited to the copayment, and the physician is precluded from charging more than the Medicare-approved amount for the service. Physicians who do not participate must collect their fee from the patient, who in turn is reimbursed by the program an amount equal to the Medicare-allowed amount for the service. If there is a difference between the physician's charge and the Medicare-allowed fee, the difference (balance billed) is subject to restrictions known as the *limiting charge*. An annual "Dear Dr." letter is sent to each physician by the Medicare carrier in his or her area giving information on the *participating approved charges, nonparticipating approved charges,* and *limiting charges* for any service for which the physician submitted Medicare claims during the previous year. The amount of the limiting charges and the decrease in the percentage of limiting charges over the years of the implementation of the program were designed to encourage physicians to become participating physicians in the Medicare program.

To Participate or Not to Participate

As a physician, you have the option of participating in Medicare. If your practice includes even a moderate number of Medicare patients, participation may help your cash flow. Because 50%–80% (depending on the service provided) of the approved Medicare fee is paid directly to you rather than to the patient, your collection process probably will be faster and accomplished with fewer administrative requirements. In addition, you may have a decided competitive edge; patients may select you because they know your participation means they have only a 20% copayment for covered services. The advantages for nonparticipation are that 1) you are able to accept assignment on a claim-by-claim basis giving you freedom of choice, which may be philosophically important to you; and 2) you are allowed to bill patients for covered services above the Medicare-approved amount (balance billing). However, there is a maximum allowable amount that you can bill in excess of the approved amount, which, since January 1933, has been 15% above the Medicare-approved amount for nonparticipating physicians (limiting charge). Offsetting that billing advantage is the fact that Medicare payments for nonparticipating physicians are 95% of payment rates for participating physicians, which effectively reduces the 15% additional billing amount to a 9.25% differential.

Medicare Physician Payment Reform

The implementation of the current Medicare physician payment system on January 1, 1992, was the result of a decade of effort by the federal government and the medical profession to alter the way Medicare paid for physician services. Pressure to change the Medicare Part B payment system increased as concerns about the escalation of Part B costs grew. In addition, the government wished to bring its Part B payment system in line with its Part A payment system, which in 1983 became a prospective payment system, using diagnosis-related groups (DRGs) as the basis for reimbursing hospitals. Since the inception of the Medicare program in 1966, physician payment had been based on a system of customary, prevailing, and reasonable charges. For almost 15 years, Medicare placed a series of controls on reimbursement levels that essentially held reimbursement to early 1970s levels. Even though there was widespread dissatisfaction with the levels of reimbursement, no substitute method for payment was considered acceptable until the development of the RBRVS.

The first relative value scale was developed by the California Medical Association in 1956, based on median charges reported by California Blue Shield. The system of payment was eventually used by a number of state Medicaid programs, Blue Cross/Blue Shield plans, and several commercial insurers to set fee schedules. However, during the late 1970s the Federal Trade Commission raised concerns about the possibility of antitrust violations, and the California Medical Association suspended the use of its relative value scale.

Under pressure to develop an alternative payment system for physician services, the Health Care Financing Administration (HCFA) turned to Hsiao and Braun (1991), two health policy research scientists at Harvard University, and funded the Harvard team to develop an RBRVS. Their work resulted in the development of a system for physician payment adopted by HCFA and the Physician Payment Review Commission of Congress and supported by the American Medical Association (AMA). In cooperating with HCFA on the development of the RBRVS system, the AMA insisted on the following features:

- Payment schedule amounts should be adjusted to reflect geographic differences in physicians' practice costs, such as office rent and wages of nonphysician personnel.
- Geographic differences in the cost of physicians' professional liability insurance would be especially important, and these differences should be reflected separately from other practice costs.
- There should be a transition period in the implementation of the system to minimize disruption in patient care and access.
- Organized medicine would seek to play a major role in updating the RBRVS.
- Physicians should have the right to decide on a claim-by-claim basis whether to accept Medicare's approved amount, including the patient's copayment, as payment in full.

The new payment reform affected all physician services. The only exceptions were physician services provided to Medicare patients enrolled in Medicare health maintenance organizations and certain services provided by teaching physicians in hospitals, skilled nursing facilities, and comprehensive outpatient rehabilitation facilities. Of interest to psychiatrists is that the payment reform also covers services provided by nurse practitioners, clinical nurse specialists, clinical psychologists, and clinical social workers.

The AMA (1996a) publishes *Medicare RBRVS: The Physicians' Guide,* which is updated every year. The book is divided into five sections: Roots of Medicare's RBRVS Payment System, Major Components of the RBRVS Payment System, RBRVS Payment System and Operation, RBRVS Payment System in Your Practice, and reference lists and appendixes. The book contains valuable information about the RBRVS program that can be applied directly to your practice. The book can be ordered by writing the

Medicare RBRVS Order Department, OP059698, American Medical Association, 515 North State Street, Chicago, Illinois, 60610, or by calling (800) 621-8335.

Medicare Payment Policies Important for Psychiatrists

Telephone Management

Payment is not made for telephone consultations. HCFA considers this pre- or postservice work.

Injections

If you provide a subcutaneous intramuscular or intravenous injection in conjunction with a patient visit, no additional payment is made for administering the injection. However, HCFA will pay for the drug injected. The identification of the drug injected is done through a Health Care Financing Administration Common Procedure Coding System (HCPC) (1998) level II code, and Table 6–1 lists the codes for injectables.

Payment for Nonphysicians

The Medicare program provides payment for clinical psychologists, clinical social workers, physician assistants (PAs), nurse practitioners, and clinical nurse specialists. These providers must be licensed or have limited licenses.

Clinical Psychologists

Clinical psychologists must meet licensing or certification standards for the state in which they practice. Licensing requires psychologists to hold a doctoral degree in psychology from a program in clinical psychology at an accredited educational institution. In addition, a psychologist must possess

Table 6–1. Injectables

Drug	Code
Amitriptyline hydrochloride (up to 20 mg)	J1320
Amobarbital (up to 125 mg)	J0300
Chlordiazepoxide hydrochloride (up to 100 mg)	J1990
Chlorpromazine hydrochloride (up to 50 mg)	J3230
Diazepam (up to 5 mg)	J3360
Fluphenazine decanoate (up to 25 mg)	J2680
Haloperidol (up to 5 mg)	J1630
Haloperidol decanoate (50 mg)	J1631
Imipramine hydrochloride (up to 25 mg)	J3270
Lorazepam (2 mg)	J2060
Perphenazine (up to 5 mg)	J3310
Prochlorperazine (up to 10 mg)	J0780
Triflupromazine hydrochloride (up to 20 mg)	J3400
Unclassified drug	J3490
Nonprescription drugs	A9150

Source. Codes are from Healthcare Financing Administration Common Procedure Coding System 1998.

2 years of supervised clinical experience, one of which is postdegree. Diagnostic tests furnished by clinical psychologists are paid under the physician payment schedule as are all other payment schedule services. Diagnostic services provided by psychologists who do not meet the requirements for a clinical psychologist are paid based on reasonable charge.

Clinical Social Workers

Clinical social workers must possess master's degrees or doctoral degrees in social work and have at least 2 years of supervised clinical social work experience. The social worker must be licensed or certified by the state in which the services are performed.

Physician Assistants

Medicare covers PA services that are provided under the supervision of a physician when the services are 1) furnished in a hospital, skilled nursing facility, or nursing facility or 2) furnished in a rural health professional shortage area. Payment for PA services provided in hospitals is limited to 75% and other covered services to 85% of the physician reimbursement. Payment is made directly to the facility where the PA services were provided.

Nurse Practitioners and Clinical Nurse Specialists

Payment for services provided by a nurse practitioner working in collaboration with a physician in a *skilled nursing facility* or in a *nursing facility* may be covered and payment made to the nurse practitioner's employer. Payment may be made directly to the nurse practitioner for services provided in a rural area other than those services provided in a hospital setting. In nursing facilities the allowed amount is 85% of the physician payment schedule. In a rural area the amount allowed will be limited to the lower actual charge or 75% of the physician payment schedule for services in a hospital and 85% of the physician payment for all other settings.

"Incident to" Services

Medicare covers services provided by a nonphysician employee that are "incident to" physician services and pays for them under the payment schedule as if a physician performed the service. Coverage of these services applies not only to nonphysician employees, such as nurses or technicians, but also to nonphysician, licensed practitioners who assist or act in the place of a physician. Originally, HCFA defined *reimbursable incident to services* narrowly (e.g., administering injections, taking blood pressures and temperatures, and changing dressings). In 1993 the definition was broadened to include services ordinarily performed by the physician, such as physical examinations, minor surgery, setting casts or simple fractures, and reading X rays. It is important that you understand this rule and not bill for services not covered by the rule (e.g., psychotherapeutic services provided by unlicensed master's-level employees). Also, when billing under your tax ID number for services provided by a clinical social worker or clinical psychologist employed by you, you must use the HCPC modifier -**AH** for clinical psychologists or -**AJ** for clinical social workers. You also have the option of obtaining personal identification numbers (PINs) for those employees (licensed psychologists and/or social workers) and billing under their PINs but receiving payment to your tax ID number. You should not bill for their services under your PIN because the carrier will assume you provided the service.

Medicare Teaching-Physician Rules

On December 8, 1995, HCFA issued new regulations revising the rules for Medicare Part B payment for services of teaching physicians. The new regulations became effective July 1, 1996.

General Rule

If a resident (or fellow) participates in a service furnished in a teaching setting, a Part B payment will be allowed only if the teaching physician is present during the key portion of any service or procedure for which payment is sought. HCFA has eliminated all current attending physician criteria. An attending physician relationship is no longer required in order to code and bill, and the term *attending physician* is replaced with *teaching physician*. Each physician will determine the *key portion* of any service or procedure furnished. This concept is intended to provide flexibility to the rule and to avoid requiring the presence of the teaching physician for the full duration of every service or procedure coded and billed in his or her name. Although HCFA understands that it may be difficult for providers to determine the key portions for a particular service, the concept is necessarily general as it is not feasible to define the key portion for all services prospectively.

Evaluation and Management Services

For evaluation and management (E/M) services, the teaching physician must be present during the portion of the service that determines the level of service coded and billed. HCFA believes that the teaching physician should have considerable discretion in determining the key portion of the service and therefore does not anticipate that carriers will deny claims submitted based on this discretion, as long as the claims are well documented. If the teaching physician cannot identify the key portion of the service, then he or she should be present for the entire service. The factors to be considered when selecting the appropriate level of E/M code are complexity of medical decision making, extent of history obtained, and extent of examination performed. The medical record must contain documentation that the teaching physician was present at the time the service was furnished.

Given the nature of the graduate medical education (GME) process in the organizational structure of psychiatric residency programs, HCFA has determined that an exception to the physical presence requirement for selected services provided in certain outpatient centers is appropriate. In late May 1996, HCFA provided written instructions to Medicare carriers regarding these exceptions for psychiatry. For procedure codes based on time (e.g., psychotherapy codes **90804–90829**), the teaching physician must be present for the period of time for which the claim is made. For example, carriers pay for a code that specifically describes a service lasting 20–30 minutes only if the teaching physician is present for 20–30 minutes. Do not add time spent by the resident in the absence of the teaching physician to time spent by the resident and teaching physician with the beneficiary or time spent by the teaching physician alone with the beneficiary. Currently, according to HCFA, this guideline means minute-for-minute physical presence or concurrent viewing by the teaching physician.

A requirement for psychiatry services furnished under an approved GME program is the presence of the teaching physician during the service or concurrent observation of the service by use of a one-way mirror or video equipment. Use of audio equipment only does not meet this exception for the physical presence requirement. Furthermore, the teacher supervising the resident must be a physician; the Medicare teaching-physician policy does not apply to psychologists who supervise psychiatric residents in approved GME programs.

Medicare Private Contracting

Under the terms of the Balanced Budget Act of 1997, effective January 1, 1998, Medicare patients may go outside the Medicare system for health care. Medicare payment rules, including limiting charges and fee schedule amounts, would not apply to any items or services furnished under private contracts. However, any physician entering into a private contract with even *one* Medicare patient is then barred from submitting *any* claims on behalf of any Medicare beneficiary for 2 years.

Questions and Answers

1. I take care of very few Medicare patients. Is there any reason for me to study and understand the RBRVS

Medicare system of payment to physicians?

The Medicare RBRVS physician payment system is now being used by many commercial carriers; therefore, you should become familiar with the payment system.

2. **If I am a nonparticipating physician (do not accept Medicare assignment), can I charge a Medicare patient my full fee for a covered service?**

Nonparticipating physicians are allowed to bill Medicare patients for covered services above the Medicare-approved amount, which is referred to as *balance billing.* However, the amount a nonparticipating physician can bill a Medicare patient in excess of the approved amount is subject to limitations. Since January 1993, the limiting charge has been 15% above the Medicare-approved amount for nonparticipating physicians. However, Medicare payments for nonparticipating physicians are 95% of payment rates for participating physicians. Therefore, the 15% limiting charge translates into only 9.25% more reimbursement than for participating physicians' charges.

3. **Are there also limiting charges for services not covered by Medicare?**

Fees for services not covered by Medicare are the responsibility of the patient. Charges should be your usual and customary charges to any patient regardless of payer status.

4. **Can I waive the deductible or copayment for an indigent patient covered by Medicare?**

The inspector general for the U.S. Department of Health and Human Services considers it fraudulent practice to routinely waive patients' Medicare copayments and deductibles. Within the current RBRVS physician payment system, if copayments and/or deductibles are routinely waived, the charge minus the copayment and/or deductible portion of the payment is considered to be the physician's actual charge. Medicare reimbursement policy dictates that payment would be the lower of either the actual charge or the approved amount. The physician must be able to demonstrate that a good faith effort was made to collect copayments and deductibles from the patient. Bills, letters, and records of telephone calls made to the patient by the physician or collection agency would provide appropriate documentation that a good faith effort was made to collect from the patient.

CHAPTER 7

Documentation

There are five excellent reasons for documenting services and procedures:

1. Documentation is good medicine. Clear, concise recording of the when, what, and why of services you provide to patients is an intrinsic component of good care. Documentation also makes clear the formulations that are the basis of treatment planning and contributes to continuity of care.
2. Documentation is the basis for selecting procedural codes. What you did for the patient is matched to the descriptors and therefore facilitates claims reviews and payment.
3. Documentation facilitates communication and continuity of care among physicians and other health professionals involved in the patient's care.

4. Documentation is your best protection against audit liability. First, documentation assists in accurate coding, which reduces the chances of an audit. Second, if you are audited, documentation is the factual data base that supports your coding and charges.
5. Documentation protects you if you are accused of malpractice because your records will support your rationale for making medical decisions and will demonstrate what, in fact, you did for the patient.

You may be convinced that documentation is a good and necessary procedure, but the specifics of documentation are less clear. What should be documented, and how much documentation is necessary? The question, How much documentation is enough? is difficult to answer, and the answer varies depending on the requirements of each insurance company. Commercial insurance companies acting as carriers for Medicare are likely to require more stringent documentation for the Medicare program than they do for their own insurance products. For documentation of evaluation and management (E/M) services, the American Medical Association (AMA) and Health Care Financing Administration (HCFA) have jointly developed a set of guidelines described in this chapter. Documentation for using the psychiatric service codes is less certain, but recent guidelines developed by the medical carriers of the Medicare program, developed in draft form by the Empire Medicare Program in New York, also are outlined in this chapter.

A review of this chapter raises realistic concerns that these elaborately defined diagnostic criteria may dictate detailed, lengthy notes to support selection of levels of E/M services and to document psychiatric services. Unfortunately, in the outpatient setting, the work associated with documentation is part of the postservice work that is already comprehended in the Relative Value Units (RVUs) for each service. However, in the inpatient setting, documentation is a component of the unit/floor time that contributes to your selection of a level of service.

The general principle to keep in mind regarding documentation is, What do payers want and why? Insurance payers must be able to demonstrate that the services for which they pay have, in fact, been performed and the services provided are consistent with the benefit package. The base information they may request includes

- The site of service
- Medical necessity and appropriateness of the diagnostic or therapeutic services provided
- Accurate reporting of services

The AMA's (1992c) published documentation principles are as follows:

- The medical record should be complete and legible.
- The documentation of each patient encounter should include the date; reason for the encounter; appropriate history and physical examination; review of laboratory, X-ray data, and other ancillary services when appropriate; assessment; and plan for care, including discharge plan if appropriate.
- Past and present diagnoses should be accessible to the treating and/or consulting physician.
- The reasons for and results of X rays, laboratory tests, and other ancillary services should be documented or included in the medical record.
- Relevant health risk factors should be identified.
- The patient's progress, including response to treatment, change in treatment, change in diagnosis, and patient noncompliance, should be documented.
- The written plan for care should include, when appropri-

ate, treatments and medications, specifying frequency and dosage; any referrals and consultations; patient/family education; and specific instructions for follow-up.

- The documentation should support the intensity of the patient evaluation and/or the treatment, including thought processes and the complexity of medical decision making.
- All entries to the medical record should be dated and authenticated.
- *Physicians' Current Procedural Terminology* (CPT)/*International Classification of Diseases,* Ninth Revision, Clinical Modification (ICD-9-CM) codes reported on the health insurance claim form or billing statement should reflect the documentation in the medical record.

Documentation Guidelines for Evaluation and Management Services

Revised guidelines were jointly published by the AMA and HCFA (CPT Assistant 1997) for E/M services with an original implementation date of July 1, 1998. Implementation has been delayed until late 1998 or early 1999. The following discussions highlight the documentation guidelines for the three key components of E/M services (history, examination, and medical decision making). To completely understand the documentation guidelines, you must review the revised guidelines of AMA and HCFA (CPT Assistant 1997), as well as the Evaluation and Management (E/M) Guidelines section of the CPT manual. The following documentation guidelines have been constructed from definitions and instructions for selecting levels of service that are in the E/M Guidelines section (American Medical Association 1997, pp. 1–8).

History

Table 7–1 illustrates the construction of a patient's history, described in *CPT Assistant* (CPT Assistant 1997).

Table 7–2 indicates the number of items required in each element of a patient's history for each of the four levels of history taking. Please note that a chief complaint is required for each level of history.

Interval review of systems (ROS) and/or past, family, and social history may be documented by describing new ROS and/or past, family, and social history or by noting there has been no change and providing the date and location of the previous ROS and past, family, and social history.

The ROS and past, family, and social history may be obtained by ancillary staff or on forms completed by the patient. The physician must review the data and document the review supplementing and/or confirming the data. By doing so, the physician takes medical-legal responsibility for the accuracy of the data.

If the condition of the patient prevents obtaining a history, the physician should describe the patient's condition or circumstances that preclude obtaining the history.

Examination

The AMA and HCFA (CPT Assistant 1997) have established single-system examinations for 11 single organ systems. Table 7–3 shows the elements of the psychiatric single-system examination.

The required number of elements for each level of examination is listed in Table 7–4.

Medical Decision Making

The last of the key factors for choosing level of service is the complexity of medical decision making, which consists of three elements and four levels outlined in Tables 7–5, 7–6,

Table 7–1.   Construction of a patient's history

Element	Description	Items
Chief complaint	A brief statement usually in the patient's own words	Symptom, problem, condition, diagnosis, reason for the encounter
History of the present illness	A chronological description of the development of the patient's present illness	Associated signs and symptoms Context Duration Location Modifying factors Quality Severity Timing
Review of systems	An inventory of body systems to identify signs and/or symptoms	Allergic, immunologic Cardiovascular Constitutional (fever, weight loss) Ears, nose, mouth, throat Endocrine Eyes Gastrointestinal Genitourinary Hematologic, lymphatic Integumentary (skin, breast) Musculoskeletal Neurologic Psychiatric Respiratory Construction of a patient's history

(continued)

Table 7–1.   Construction of a patient's history *(continued)*

Element	Description	Items
Past, family, and/or social history	A chronological review of relevant data	Past history: illnesses, operations, injuries, treatments Family history: family medical history, events, hereditary illnesses Social history: age-appropriate review of past and current activities

7–7, and 7–8. The documentation requirements for deciding the level of complexity are not as specific as they are for the history and examination. In Tables 7–5 through 7–8, I attempt to illustrate by examples the three elements of medical decision making. To qualify for a given type of decision making, two of the three elements in Table 7–5 must be met or exceeded.

Time

Time as a component in selecting the level of service has been defined and discussed in Chapter 4. Table 7–9 is an example of an auditor's work sheet for making the decision to use time in selecting the level of service. The three questions are prompts that assist the auditor (usually a nurse reviewer) in assessing if the clinician 1) documented the length of time of the patient encounter, 2) described the counseling or coordination of care, and 3) indicated more than half of the encounter time was for counseling or coordination of care.

Table 7–2. Required elements for choosing level of history

History elements	Problem focused	Expanded problem focused	Detailed	Comprehensive
History of present illness				
Associated signs and symptoms	Brief (1–3 elements)	Brief (1–3 elements)	Extended (4 or more elements)	Extended (4 or more elements)
Context				
Duration				
Location				
Modifying factors				
Quality				
Severity				
Timing				
Review of systems				
Allergic, immunologic	None	Pertinent to problem (1 system)	Extended (2–9 systems)	Complete (10 or more systems, or some systems with statement "all others negative")
Cardiovascular				
Constitutional (fever, weight loss)				
Ears, nose, mouth, throat				
Endocrine				
Eyes				
Gastrointestinal				

	None	None	Pertinent (1 history area)	Complete (2 or 3 history areas)
Genitourinary				
Hematologic, lymphatic				
Integumentary (skin, breast)				
Musculoskeletal				
Neurologic				
Psychiatric				
Respiratory				
All others negative	None			
Past medical, family, social history		None		
Past history (patient's past experiences with illnesses, operations, injuries, and treatments)				
Family history (review of medical events in the patient's family, including diseases that may be hereditary or may place the patient at risk)				
Social history (age-appropriate review of past and current activities)				

Table 7–3.   Psychiatric examination

System/body area	Elements of examination
Constitutional	• Measurement of any *three* of the following *seven* vital signs: 1) sitting or standing blood pressure, 2) supine blood pressure, 3) pulse rate and regularity, 4) respiration, 5) temperature, 6) height, and 7) weight (may be measured and recorded by ancillary staff)
	• General appearance of patient (e.g., development, nutrition, body habitus, deformities, attention to grooming)
Musculoskeletal	• Assessment of muscle strength and tone (e.g., flaccid, cogwheel, spastic), with notation of any atrophy and abnormal movements
	• Examination of gait and station
Psychiatric	• Description of speech, including rate, volume, articulation, coherence, and spontaneity, with notation of abnormalities (e.g., perseveration, paucity of language)
	• Description of thought processes, including rate of thoughts, content of thoughts (e.g., logical versus illogical, tangential), abstract reasoning, and computation
	• Description of associations (e.g., loose, tangential, circumstantial, intact)
	• Description of abnormal psychotic thoughts, including hallucinations, delusions, preoccupation with violence, homicidal or suicidal ideation, and obsessions

(continued)

- Description of the patient's judgment (e.g., concerning everyday activities and social situations) and insight (e.g., concerning psychiatric condition)
- Complete mental status examination, including
  - Orientation to time, place, and person
  - Recent and remote memory
  - Attention span and concentration
  - Language (e.g., naming objects, repeating phrases)
  - Fund of knowledge (e.g., awareness of current events, past history, vocabulary)
  - Mood and affect (e.g., depression, anxiety, agitation, hypomania, lability)

Table 7–4.   Content and documentation requirements

Level of examination	Elements of examination[a]
Problem focused	One to five elements identified by a bullet
Expanded problem focused	At least six elements identified by a bullet
Detailed	At least nine elements identified by a bullet
Comprehensive	Perform all elements identified by a bullet

[a]See Table 7–3 for bulleted lists.

Revised Evaluation and Management Documentation Guidelines

Following the AMA/HCFA publication of the revised Evaluation and Management Documentation Guidelines in July 1997, the many comments received by the AMA from components of organized medicine and others resulted in a delay of implementation by HCFA and new framework for documentation guidelines developed by a work group of the CPT Editorial Panel supported by AMA and HCFA staff. This new framework is offered as a work in progress that will receive extensive review, refinement, and revision by all components of organized medicine before new guidelines are available for pilot testing. The proposed changes will most likely include the following:

- Shorten the document substantially.
- Emphasize that a code may be selected and documented based on *counseling/coordination of care time alone,* without reference needed to any other dimensions of code selection (i.e., history, examination, complexity of medical decision making).
- Emphasize that, for established patients, only *two of three*

Table 7–5. Elements of medical decision making

Number of diagnoses or management options[a]	Amount and/or complexity of data to be reviewed[b]	Risk of complications and/or morbidity or mortality[c]	Type of decision making
Minimal	Minimal or none	Minimal	Straight-forward
Limited	Limited	Low	Low complexity
Multiple	Moderate	Moderate	Moderate complexity
Extensive	Extensive	High	High complexity

[a]See Table 7–6. [b]See Table 7–7. [c]See Table 7–8.
Source. Adapted from CPT Assistant 1997.

history areas (history of present illness [HPI], ROS, and past family and/or social history [PFSH]) instead of *all three* need to be documented.

- Add a clear note that, when a history cannot be obtained because of specific patient conditions (e.g., inability to communicate urgent, emergent situation), the history is deemed "comprehensive" for coding and documentation purposes.
- Simplify examination criteria and enhance their clinical flexibility by eliminating forced and artificial distinctions between general multisystem exams and single-system exams and eliminating confusing shaded and unshaded boxes.
- Eliminate confusing examination instructions that take the form of "perform all elements and document two elements."
- Simplify the medical decision-making section by eliminating one level (low complexity)—the proposed levels are straightforward, moderate, and high complexity.

Table 7–6. Number of diagnoses or management options

	Minimal	Limited	Multiple	Extensive
Diagnoses	1 Established	1 Established 1 Rule out *or* Differential	2 Rule out *or* Differential	> 2 Rule out *or* Differential
Problem(s)	Improved Controlled Resolved	Stable Resolving	Unstable Failing to change	Worsening marked change
Management options[a]	1 or 2	2 or 3	3 or more changes in treatment plan	4 or more changes in treatment plan

Note. The highest level in any one category determines the overall level.
[a]For example, patient instructions, nursing instructions, therapies, medications, referrals, and consultations.

Table 7–7. Amount and/or complexity of data to be reviewed

	Minimal	Limited	Multiple	Extensive
Medical data	1 source	2 sources	3 sources	Multiple sources
Diagnostic tests	2	3	4	> 4
Review of results	Confirmatory review	Confirmation of results with another physician	Results discussed with physician performing tests	Unexpected results, contradictory reviews, requires additional reviews

Note. The highest level in any one category determines the overall level.

Table 7–8. Risk of complications and/or morbidity or mortality

Level of risk	Presenting problem(s)	Diagnostic procedure(s) ordered	Management options selected
Minimal	• One self-limited or minor problem (e.g., medication side effect)	• Laboratory tests requiring venipuncture • ECG/EEG • Urinalysis	• Reassurance
Low	• Two or more self-limited or minor problems • One stable chronic illness (e.g., well-controlled depression) • Acute uncomplicated illness (e.g., exacerbation of anxiety disorder)	• Psychological testing • Skull film • CT/MRI • Neuropsychological testing	• Psychotherapy • Environmental intervention; agency schools, vocational • Referral for consultation; physician, social work
Moderate	• One or more chronic illnesses with mild exacerbation, progression, or side effects of treatment	• Obtain fluid from the body (e.g., lumbar puncture)	• Prescription drug management • Open-door seclusion

	• Two or more stable chronic illnesses	• ECT, inpatient, outpatient, routine; no comorbid medical conditions
	• (Undiagnosed new problem with uncertain prognosis (e.g., psychosis)	
High	• One or more chronic illnesses with severe exacerbation, progression, or side effect of treatment (e.g., schizophrenia)	• Drug therapy requiring intensive monitoring (e.g., Valium taper for withdrawal patient)
	• Acute or chronic illness with threat to life (e.g., suicidal or homicidal ideation)	• Closed-door seclusion
		• Suicide observation
	• An abrupt change in mental status (e.g., delirium)	• ECT; patient has comorbid medical condition (e.g., cardiovascular disease)
		• Rapid IM neuroleptic administration
		• Pharmacologic restraint (e.g., Inapsine)

Note. The highest level in any one category determines the overall level. ECG = electrocardiogram; EEG = electroencephalogram; CT = computed tomography; MRI = magnetic resonance imaging; ECT = electroconvulsive therapy; IM = intramuscular.

Table 7–9.   Choosing level based on time

Does documentation reveal total time?	Yes	No
Time: Face-to-face in outpatient setting Unit/floor in inpatient setting		
Does documentation describe the content of counseling or coordinating care?	Yes	No
Does documentation suggest that more than half of time was counseling or coordinating care?	Yes	No
If all answers are *yes,* select level based on time.		

Note.   If the physician documents total time and suggests that counseling or coordinating care dominates (more than 50%) the encounter, time may determine level of service. Documentation may refer to prognosis, differential diagnosis, risks, benefits of treatment, instructions, compliance, risk reduction, or discussion with another health care provider.

- Further simplify the medical decision-making section by allowing the highest complexity element (i.e., the number of diagnoses/risk of complications, diagnostic procedures/tests and/or data to be reviewed or management options) to drive selection of the level of decision making. This change eliminates the need to make a separate selection from the table of risk and then entering that decision into another matrix.

Psychiatric Diagnostic and Therapeutic Procedures

Currently, there are no universal, standardized documentation guidelines for psychiatric diagnostic and therapeutic procedures (CPT codes **90801–90889**) similar to the documentation guidelines for E/M codes presented in this chapter. Documentation guidelines for psychiatric diagnostic and therapeutic procedures have been published by several Medicare carriers (e.g., Xact, Empire Medical Services, Blue

Cross/Blue Shield of Texas) in conjunction with coding guidelines, benefit descriptions, and payment policies. In the following discussions, I present a consolidated version of these documentation requirements.

General Clinical Psychiatric
Diagnostic or Evaluative Procedure—90801

A general clinical psychiatric diagnostic or evaluative procedure is similar in work effort to level III initial hospital care (99223), which requires a comprehensive history, a comprehensive examination, and high-complexity medical decision making. In fact, Medicare will allow physicians to use either 99223 or 90801 for the first hospital day. Outpatient consultations (99243, 99244) and inpatient consultations (99253, 99254) are also equivalent in work effort to code 90801.

The elements of a diagnostic evaluation (90801) suggested by Medicare carriers, although not organized as key factors, are the following:

- Chief complaint
- Referral source
- History of present illness (HPI)
- Past psychiatric history
- Past medical history
- Social and family history
- Mental status examination
- Strengths and liabilities
- Multiaxis diagnoses
- Treatment plan

Interactive Psychiatric Diagnostic
Interview Examination—90802

The elements of an interactive psychiatric diagnostic interview examination are identical to those previously listed for code **90801**. However, the work effort is increased because of the patient's inability to communicate with the evaluator through normal verbal communication. In addition to the elements previously listed for code **90801**, documentation must include the fact that the patient does not have the ability to interact with the evaluator through normal verbal communication.

Psychiatric Therapeutic Procedures

Codes for psychiatric therapeutic procedures include **90865** (narcosynthesis), **90804–90829** (individual psychotherapy), **90845** (psychoanalysis), **90846** (family psychotherapy), **90847** (conjoint family psychotherapy), **90849** (multiple-family group psychotherapy), **90853** (group psychotherapy), and **90857** (interactive group psychotherapy).

General Documentation Guidelines for Psychiatric Therapeutic Procedures

General documentation guidelines for psychiatric therapeutic procedures are the following:

- Date of service
- Time spent for the encounter
- Documentation of therapeutic intervention (insight, support, behavior modification, interactive)
- Patient's response to intervention
- Target symptoms and progress of achievement of treatment goals
- Diagnoses
- Legible signature

Special Documentation Gidelines for Psychiatric Therapeutic Procedures

There are a number of special documentation guidelines for some of the psychiatric therapeutic procedures.

Narcosynthesis (90865). Document the rationale for us-ing this procedure (e.g., relaxation and removal of inhibi-tions to discuss difficult material).

Individual psychotherapy (90804–90829). Document the site of service (i.e., inpatient or outpatient facility) and list any E/M services provided. According to HCFA, medical E/M services include the following nonexhaustive list: medi-cal diagnostic evaluation, drug management (when indi-cated), physician orders, and interpretation of laboratory or other medical diagnostic studies or observations.

Psychoanalysis (90845). Document the general guide-lines, as listed earlier, plus analytic techniques used.

Interactive group psychotherapy (90857). Document the medical necessity for using this code (i.e., the patients' minimal verbal communication skills and inability to inter-act with the therapist).

Central Nervous System Assessments/Tests

Neurocognitive, mental status, speech testing (96100, 96105, 96110, 96111, 96115, 96117). Documenta-tion guidelines include date of service, time of service, evalu-ation that determines the need for and types of testing, previous testing (tests administered, scoring, and interpreta-tion), current tests administered, scoring, interpretations, treatment recommendations, diagnoses, and legible signature.

Questions and Answers

1. This chapter apparently suggests different documen-tation requirements for different sets of codes (E/M

versus psychiatric evaluation and procedures) and different payers (Medicare versus commercial). Does this mean I have to tailor my patient records and notes to these various sets of documentation requirements?

You need to be aware of these various sets of documentation requirements (as they evolve) so that you develop a record-keeping system that is tailored to your practice. For example, if your practice is office based and you use CPT psychiatric evaluation and procedure codes almost exclusively, your records will not include the documentation methodology necessary for using the E/M codes. If your practice includes hospital services and you use E/M hospital service codes, your hospital records will include the documentation requirements associated with E/M hospital service codes.

2. **Is it necessary for the physician to record the examination himself or herself, or can a patient checklist be used?**

A checklist would be acceptable if there is a narrative report of the important positive and relevant negative findings. Abnormal findings should be described. A notation of *abnormal* without a description would not be sufficient.

3. **How much detail is required in recording the ROS for the various levels of the patient's history?**

The following information is required:

- *Problem-pertinent system review:* Positive and negative questions and responses directly related to the problem(s) may be incorporated in the HPI and do not have to be recorded separately a second time as an ROS.

- *Extended system review:* The problem-related ROS would be recorded as described earlier, and the review of additional systems also should be listed in the HPI. Notations indicating the positives and negatives (e.g., cardiovascular-negative) would be sufficient.
- *Complete system review:* In the HPI, at least 10 of the following systems must be addressed by the ROS. A single-statement ROS-negative is not sufficient; notation of specific system negatives (e.g., cardiovascular-negative) is sufficient. In addition, if there is a current ROS in the chart, reference to that ROS may suffice.

- Allergic-immunologic
- Cardiovascular
- Ears, nose, mouth, and throat
- Endocrine
- Eyes
- Gastrointestinal
- Genitourinary
- Hematologic, lymphatic
- Integumentary (skin, breast)
- Musculoskeletal
- Neurologic
- Psychiatric
- Respiratory

4. **Is it necessary for the physician himself or herself to record the ROS and the family and social history?**
No. Various methods of collecting the data are acceptable, provided there is documentation that the physician reviewed the data and incorporated the data into his or her medical decision making.

Acceptable documentation includes the following:

- A notation such as *reviewed* with date and signature
- Comments written to clarify information, with date and signature
- Comments written in the narrative of the progress note or consultation report that clarify or expand on information obtained from the alternative source, with date and signature

5. **Does the answer to question 4 include ROS and family and social history data obtained from forms or checklists filled out by the patient?**

   Yes, but the physician is responsible for the accuracy of the data and must indicate his or her review of the data by noting *reviewed* with date and signature.

CHAPTER 8

Putting It All Together for Accurate Coding

By the time you have reached this chapter, I hope you have been convinced that accurate coding and appropriate documentation are essential for supporting the billing and collection functions of your practice. The availability of *Physicians' Current Procedural Terminology* (CPT) coding, diagnostic coding systems (*Diagnostic and Statistical Manual of Mental Disorders,* Fourth Edition [DSM-IV]/*International Classification of Diseases, Ninth Revision, Clinical Modification* [ICD-9-CM]), and current information technology has enabled commercial insurance companies, managed care organizations, and the federal government (Health Care Financing Administration [HCFA]) to create data bases of physician charging activity that can be easily retrieved and analyzed in many different ways. These data bases are being used to monitor and audit physician practices to achieve the payers' goals of efficient utilization of treatment resources. These capabilities have contributed to changes in the medical marketplace and have created many new challenges for clinicians.

Information technologies are a permanent part of the medical landscape. We must learn to cope with this reality and to use constructively the products of technology to improve patient care and protect the financial basis of our practices. The bottom-line message is that the business aspects of your practice must be precise to ensure you are appropriately reimbursed for your services. Coding should be accurate: time spent resubmitting claims or resolving claim disputes will result in lost dollars; do it right the first time. In this chapter I will summarize the guide to coding and documentation that will assist you in filing claims accurately and efficiently.

Step 1.   Identify and Record Every Service You Provide

You are probably proficient in recording commonly performed services such as new patient evaluations, psychotherapy sessions, and hospital visits. The fewer the kinds of services and procedures you provide patients, the easier it is to track and record those services and procedures. For example, recording the services in an office practice with patients scheduled for x number of hours per day and y number of days per week is a straightforward process. But psychiatric practices offer more complex, multiple services at various sites (e.g., in the office, hospital, day hospital, emergency room), with varying levels and times of service. If you rely on your memory at the end of the day to tally up all of the services you have provided at the various service sites, you may forget some billable services. Make a list of the services, codes, and diagnoses you use most frequently to save time. **Keep a notebook and record every service immediately after the service is provided.**

You probably provide services to patients every day that you may not think of as worthy of being recorded for eventual billing (e.g., making telephone calls, writing reports and letters, providing educational supplies and patient information, incurring unusual travel costs). Considering the persistent, downward pressure on physician reimbursement, you may have to reconsider charging for these services. If you do so, you must discipline yourself to record these services as systematically as you record the more commonly provided services.

Step 2. Document Your Services

The guidelines and recommendations for documenting services are covered in Chapter 7. However, the following examples may help you structure your medical notes.

Guidelines for Inpatient Attending Progress Note

The guidelines for an inpatient attending progress note are as follows:

- Date
- Interval history
- Mental status examination (symptomatology to support DSM-IV diagnosis)

- Discussion of medical decision making
  - Progress toward achieving treatment plan
  - Changes in treatment plan
  - Medication response, side effects, and/or changes
  - Ordering/reviewing test results and/or consultations
  - Updating length of stay
  - Plans for aftercare
- Staff and/or team meeting reports
- Other counseling/coordination of care
- Total unit/floor time
- Signature

The following is an example of an inpatient attending progress note:

9/20/96 Attending Note

Mr. Smith reported he was feeling less depressed. He was alert, cooperative, and oriented in three spheres. He exhibited no delusional thinking and no suicidal thinking. There was no evidence of extrapyramidal symptoms. He complained of a dry mouth.

- History (problem focused)
- Examination (problem-focused mental status examination)

Time: 5 minutes

Note continues:

Will maintain current doses of antidepressants and neuroleptics. Suggest fluids be made available for dry mouth. Nursing note indicates improved mood, affect stable, patient participating in ward activities. Thyroid studies are normal.

- Medical decision making (straightforward; review of the nurse's notes plus charting the progress notes and review of test results)

Time: 5 minutes

Total time: 10 minutes unit/floor time

Signature

Code recommended:

99231   Subsequent hospital care

But if the nursing notes had indicated the patient was "cheeking" medications, the following work might be required:

- Coordination of care: meeting with primary nurse to discuss patient's noncompliance, meeting with treatment team to develop treatment strategy, incorporating strategy in treatment plan

Time: 10 minutes

- Counseling: return to patient to confront patient about noncompliance and provide education about medications

Time: 5 minutes

Time: 3 key factors, 10 minutes

Coordination of care and counseling: 15 minutes

Total time: 25 minutes

Signature

Code recommended:

99232   Subsequent hospital care

Basis for selection of level of care: coordination of care and counseling was more than 50% of the unit/floor time

Guidelines for Outpatient Progress Note

The guidelines for an outpatient progress note are as follows:

- Date
- Interval history
- Mental status examination (symptomatology to support DSM-IV diagnosis)
- Description of psychotherapeutic process
- Discussion of medical decision making
  - Progress toward achieving treatment plan
  - Changes in treatment plan
  - Medication response, side effects, and/or changes
  - Ordering/reviewing test results and/or consultations
  - Updating number of future visits
- Total time of session
- Signature

The following is an example of an outpatient progress note:

9/20/96 Progress Note

Since last session 1 week ago, Mr. Smith reports he is feeling slightly more depressed. His job search has not gone well. He is well groomed, alert, cooperative; mild speech latency, mood moderately depressed. No suicidal ideation. He has been compliant with medications (Prozac 40 mg qhs); no side effects. I will maintain the current dose. Psychotherapeutic process focused on his procrastination in initiating job interviews and his anger toward his wife for her pressure. He acknowledges the legitimacy of his wife's concerns but reacts to her in a manner similar to his response to his mother pushing him to do better in school during his high-school and college years. Estimated number of sessions: minimally 10 to stabilize depression and work through the above psychotherapeutic issues.

Time: 45 minutes

Signature

Step 3.   Select a Code

The basic principle in selecting a code is *select the code that most accurately reflects the service or procedure you provided to your patient.*

If your practice is office based and your services consist mostly of psychiatric evaluation and therapeutic procedures, you will be using codes **90801–90899** (American Medical Association [AMA] 1997, pp. 351–354). In CPT 98, the revisions for this section are extensive (see Chapter 3 in this handbook). Be sure to review the new text, codes, and number changes for "old" codes. Once you become familiar with all the changes, you should not have problems matching procedures to codes.

Codes **90882–90899** cover a variety of services: environmental intervention for medical management, evaluation of hospital records, interpretation of results, preparation of reports, and unlisted services. These services are increasingly important in the era of managed care and accurately reflect much of the non-face-to-face work we must do on the patient's behalf. However, Medicare and an increasing number of commercial insurers will not reimburse us for these services. Nevertheless, when these services are provided distinctly from the evaluation and management (E/M) services provided in conjunction with individual psychotherapy, they can be coded and billed.

E/M codes will be used by those of you who care for patients in hospital or partial hospital settings (**99221–99239**), provide inpatient consultations (**99251–99263**), and/or provide patient services in nursing facilities (**99321–99333**). Home services are covered by codes **99341–99350**. The guidelines for selecting the level of service for E/M codes are described in Chapter 4.

Step 4.   Submit the Claim

Recall from Chapter 5 the description of claims processing and the personnel involved. The following suggestions also will help in the claims submission process:

- Claim forms must be filled out completely and legibly. Do not give the carrier a reason to return your claim; carriers take long enough to process clean claim forms. Time is money in the billing process.
- Send daily charges on each patient on separate forms. Although separate forms take slightly more time to complete, forms with multiple dates of services are easy targets for delay or return.
- Consider electronic submission of claims because you will bypass both the carrier mail room and claims examiners, thereby eliminating two sources of potential delay in the processing of your claims.
- If you submit a claim for an unusual service or use a code that has a modifier, include a brief explanatory note (see Chapter 3).

- Insurance companies now use sophisticated claims review software that includes clinical edits for CPT and ICD-9-CM codes to process claims. Billing data flagged by these software edits are subject to special review, often resulting in rejection of the claims or requests for additional information about the claims. In either instance, payment is delayed. Andrea L. Albaum-Feinstein, M.D.A., R.R.A. (1996), has developed a list of these edits. Being aware of the following edits may save you both time and money.

  - Verify official CPT and ICD-9-CM codes and descriptions. Claims review software makes it essential that clinicians are aware of annual coding updates (e.g., in CPT 98, the codes for individual psychotherapy underwent substantial changes). Because ICD-9-CM is recognized as the universal coding system for billing purposes, the few discrepancies between DSM-IV and ICD-9-CM codes occasionally may cause problems in such software. The DSM-IV to ICD-9-CM crosswalk (American Psychiatric Association 1994) can help clinicians identify such potential compatibility problems.
  - Verify clinical appropriateness of the ICD-9-CM code or diagnosis with the CPT code or procedure (e.g., a psychiatric diagnosis is not expected with a surgical procedure code).
  - Verify clinical appropriateness of the physician's specialty (e.g., a psychiatrist is not expected to be performing surgery).
  - Verify clinical appropriateness of the patient's sex and age for the diagnosis and procedure (e.g., a male is not expected to have a diagnosis of pregnancy or a child to be given electroconvulsive therapy).

- Verify the CPT code for *unlisted service.* An explanation for the use of this code and a description of the service should always accompany the claim.
- Verify the codes that insurance companies consider nonpayable. These codes vary according to the benefits policies of insurance companies. Examples might include CPT codes for telephone calls or cosmetic surgery.
- Verify appropriateness of CPT category/subcategory service codes and other E/M codes (e.g., if a clinician submits the code for an initial outpatient visit for a patient at the beginning of each year, the computer would automatically code this service as an established patient visit).
- Verify appropriateness of the charge for a specific CPT code. Each insurance company has a range of values for payment based on the specific CPT procedural code. If the range for a service is between $75 and $100 and the clinician bills $200, the claim would be flagged.
- Select CPT codes that do not conflict with coding instructions (e.g., billing for both **90801**, psychiatric diagnostic interview examination, and **99221**, initial hospital evaluation).
- Verify bundling or unbundling CPT codes to maximize reimbursement. *Bundling* is the practice of combining several procedures or services into one code when these services should be billed separately. *Unbundling* is the practice of billing for separate codes when one code for combined services should be used.
- Select claims by clinician, specialty, age, sex, or diagnostic or procedural codes for quality assurance or utilization audits.

Summary

As you code your claims, keep in mind the following suggestions:

- Make coding a priority for the business component of your practice. The coding process affects your reimbursement, and proper coding prevents audits.
- Buy and read the CPT manual published annually by the AMA.
- Keep in touch with your colleagues through the insurance committee of your district branch of the American Psychiatric Association (APA) about coding and billing issues.
- Use codes appropriately; medical fraud is the number two priority of the U.S. Justice Department.
- Code and bill for all services that you provide to patients regardless of local and/or national payer policies. The developing data base of physician charges eventually may help practitioners change payment policies for more favorable reimbursement of mental health services.

Questions and Answers

1. **Codes and documentation keep changing. How can I keep up with the changes to be sure I am coding and documenting properly?**

   Because the CPT Editorial Panel adds and modifies codes every year, you should obtain an updated version of CPT each year. In addition, the Work Group on Codes and Reimbursements and the Office of Economic Affairs and Practice Management are available to assist you in answering specific coding questions. Because documentation requirements follow the additions or modifications codes, these same contacts would be helpful to you in tracking the evolution of the documentation requirements.

2. **I have continuous reimbursement problems with commercial payers/Medicare carriers/medical care organizations. What can I do?**
    There are a number of steps you can take:

    - Make sure all of your insurance forms are filled out accurately, completely, and legibly. If you have attachments to the insurance form, stamp or write on attachments "please do not separate attachments."
    - Contact your local psychiatric society. The district branch can put you in touch with colleagues who have similar problems, assist you in assessing APA resources, sponsor legislation, and organize and sponsor legal actions.
    - Ask your patients for assistance. Informing patients about your problems with their insurance companies is not unethical. Patients can help by talking to their employers' human resources departments and requesting reviews of their claims.
    - Call the APA's Office of Economic Affairs and Practice Management at 1-202-682-6212. Staff members have access to a wide range of resources to help you with third-party payers.

3. **When I have questions about Medicare's reimbursement policies, whom should I call?**
    Because Medicare is administered regionally by independently contracted carriers and because each carrier establishes some of its own reimbursement policies, you should contact your local Medicare carrier directly for information on reimbursement policies that affect your

practice. The APA's Medicare Carrier Advisory Committee Network can assist you in establishing contact with the right people at your carrier. In addition, you may call the Office of Economic Affairs and Practice Management at (202) 682-6212.

APPENDIX 1

Medicare Part B Carriers

At times it may be necessary to communicate directly with the appropriate Medicare carrier within a state for answers on physician payment policy, patment procedure, or payment for a specific claim. Remember, unless the contact involves simply checking on the status of a claim, it may be advantageous to communicate with the carrier in writing to establish a written record of the request.

The Health Care Financing Administration (HCFA) of the Department of Health and Human Services compiles information on carrier names, addresses, and telephone numbers. HCFA updates this material annually to reflect any changes. State medical societies or HCFA regional offices should be able to provide updated carrier information within their regions.

Alabama
Medicare B
Blue Cross/Blue Shield of
Alabama
450 Riverchase Parkway
East Birmingham, AL
35298
(205) 988-2100
(205) 733-7255 Fax

Alaska
Medicare B
Blue Cross/Blue Shield of
North Dakota
4510 13th Avenue, S.W.
Fargo, ND 58121
(701) 282-1100
(701) 282-1002 Fax

American Samoa
Medicare B
Blue Cross/Blue Shield of
North Dakota
4510 13th Avenue, S.W.
Fargo, ND 58121
(701) 282-1100
(701) 282-1002 Fax

Arizona
Medicare B
Blue Cross/Blue Shield of
North Dakota
4510 13th Avenue, S.W.
Fargo, ND 58121
(701) 282-1100
(701) 282-1002 Fax

Arkansas
Medicare B
Arkansas Blue Cross/Blue

Shield
601 Gaines St.
Little Rock, AR 72203
(501) 378-2000
(501) 378-2804 Fax

California
Medicare B
State of California (North)
National Heritage Insurance
Company
5400 Legacy Drive
H3-3A-05
Plano, TX 75024
(916) 896-7025
(916) 896-7182 Fax
State of California (South)
Transamerica Occidental Life
Insurance Company
Medicare Operations
P.O. Box 54905
Los Angeles, CA 90054-0905
(213) 748-2311
(213) 741-6803 Fax

Colorado
Medicare B
Blue Cross/Blue Shield of
North Dakota
4510 13th Avenue, S.W.
Fargo, ND 58121
(701) 282-1100
(701) 282-1002 Fax

Connecticut
Medicare B
Metrahealth Insurance
Company
450 Columbus
Boulevard—5GB

P.O. Box 15045
Hartford, CT 06115-0450
(860) 702-6668
(860) 702-6587 Fax

Delaware
Medicare B
Medical Service Association of
Pennsylvania
P.O. Box 890065
Camp Hill, PA 17089-0065
(717) 763-3151
(717) 975-7045 Fax

District of Columbia
Medicare B
Medical Services Association of
Pennsylvania
P.O. Box 890065
Camp Hill, PA 17089-0065
(717) 763-3151
(717) 975-7045 Fax

Florida
Medicare B
Blue Cross/Blue Shield of
Florida, Inc.
532 Riverside Avenue
P.O. Box 2078
Jacksonville, FL 32231-0048
(904) 791-8155
(904) 791-8378 Fax

Georgia
Medicare B
Blue Cross/Blue Shield of
Alabama
450 Riverchase Parkway, East
Birmingham, AL 35298
(205) 988-2100

(205) 733-7255 Fax

**Guam and Northern Mariana
Islands**
Medicare B
Blue Cross/Blue Shield of
North Dakota
4510 13th Avenue, S.W.
Fargo, ND 58121
(701) 282-1100
(701) 282-1002 Fax

Hawaii
Medicare B
Blue Cross/Blue Shield of
North Dakota
4510 13th Avenue, S.W.
Fargo, ND 58121
(701) 282-1100
(701) 282-1002 Fax

Idaho
Medicare B
Connecticut General Life
Insurance Company (CGLIC)
Hartford, CT 06152
(615) 782-4576
(615) 244-6242 Fax

Illinois
Medicare B
Health Care Service
Corporation
233 North Michigan Avenue
Chicago, IL 60601
(312) 938-8000
(312) 861-0319 Fax

Indiana
Medicare B

Administar Federal, Inc.
8115 Knue Street
Indianapolis, IN 46250-2804
(317) 841-4400
(317) 841-4691 Fax

Iowa
Medicare B
IASD Health Services Corp.
636 Grand Avenue, Station 28
Des Moines, IA 50309
(515) 245-4618
(515) 245-3984 Fax

Kansas
Medicare B
Blue Cross/Blue Shield of
Kansas, Inc.
1133 Topeka Avenue
Topeka, KS 66601
(913) 291-7000
(913) 291-8532 Fax

Kentucky
Medicare B
Administar Federal, Inc.
8115 Knue Street
Indianapolis, IN 46250-2804
(317) 841-4400
(317) 841-4691 Fax

Louisiana
Medicare B
Arkansas Blue Cross/Blue
Shield
601 Gaines Street
Little Rock, AR 72203
(501) 378-2000
(501) 378-2804 Fax

Maine
Medicare B
Blue Cross/Blue Shield of
Massachusetts, Inc.
100 Summer Street
Boston, MA 02110
(617) 741-3122
(617) 741-3211 Fax

Maryland
Medicare B
Blue Cross/Blue Shield of
Texas, Inc.
P.O. Box 660156
Dallas, TX 75266-0156
(214) 766-6900
(214) 766-7612 Fax
Counties of Montgomery,
Prince Georges
Medical Service Association of
Pennsylvania
P.O. Box 890065
Camp Hill, PA 17089-0065
(717) 763-3151
(717) 975-7045 Fax

Massachusetts
Medicare B
Blue Cross/Blue Shield of
Massachusetts, Inc.
100 Summer Street
Boston, MA 02110
(617) 741-3122
(617) 741-3211 Fax

Michigan
Medicare B
Health Care Service Corp.
233 N. Michigan Avenue

Chicago, IL 60601
(312) 938-6360
(312) 861-0319 Fax

Minnesota
Medicare B
Metrahealth Insurance
Company
450 Columbus
Boulevard—5GB
P.O. Box 15045
Hartford, CT 06115-0450
(860) 702-6668
(860) 702-6587 Fax

Mississippi
Medicare B
Metrahealth Insurance
Company
450 Columbus
Boulevard—5GB
P.O. Box 15045
Hartford, CT 06115-0450
(860) 702-6668
(860) 702-6587 Fax

Missouri
Medicare B (Western Missouri)
Blue Cross/Blue Shield of
Kansas Inc.
1133 Topeka Avenue
P.O. Box 239
Topeka, KS 66601
(913) 291-7000
(913) 291-7824 Fax
Medicare B (Eastern Missouri)
General American Life
Insurance Company
P.O. Box 505
St. Louis, MO 63166

(314) 525-5441
(314) 525-5593 Fax

Montana
Medicare B
Blue Cross/Blue Shield of
Montana, Inc.
P.O. Box 4310
2501 Beltview
Helena, MT 59601
(406) 791-4000
(406) 442-9968 Fax

Nebraska
Medicare B
Blue Cross/Blue Shield of
Kansas, Inc.
1133 Topeka Avenue
P.O. Box 239
Topeka, KS 66601
(913) 291-7000
(913) 291-7824 Fax

Nevada
Medicare B
Blue Cross/Blue Shield of
North Dakota
4510 13th Avenue, S.W.
Fargo, ND 58121
(701) 282-1100
(701) 282-1002 Fax

New Hampshire
Medicare B
Blue Cross/Blue Shield of
Massachusetts Inc.
100 Summer Street
Boston, MA 02110
(617) 956-3445
(617) 350-4555 Fax

New Jersey
Medicare B
Medical Services Association of
Pennsylvania
P.O. Box 890065
Camp Hill, PA 17089-0065
(717) 763-3151
(717) 975-7045 Fax

New Mexico
Medicare B
Arkansas Blue Cross/Blue
Shield
601 Gaines Street
Little Rock, AR 72203
(501) 378-2000
(501) 378-2804 Fax

New York
Medicare B
Blue Cross/Blue Shield of
Western New York, Inc.
7-9 Court Street
Binghamton, NY 13901-3197
(716) 887-6900
(716) 887-8548 Fax
Counties of: Bronx, Columbia,
Delaware, Dutchess, Greene,
Kings, New York, Orange,
Putnam, Rockland, Suffolk,
Sullivan, Ulster, Westchester
Medicare B
Empire Blue Cross/Blue Shield
622 Third Avenue
New York, NY 10017
(212) 476-1000
(212) 682-5746 Fax

North Carolina
Medicare B
Connecticut General Life
Insurance Company (CGLIC)
Hartford, CT 06152
(615) 782-4576
(615) 244-6242 Fax

North Dakota
Medicare B
Blue Cross/Blue Shield of
North Dakota
4510 13th Avenue, S.W.
Fargo, ND 58121
(701) 282-1100
(701) 282-1002 Fax

Ohio
Medicare B
Nationwide Mutual Insurance
Company
P.O. Box 16788 or 16781
Columbus, OH 43216
(614) 249-7111
(614) 249-3732 Fax

Oklahoma
Medicare B
Arkansas Blue Cross/Blue
Shield
601 Gaines Street
Little Rock, AR 72203
(501) 378-2000
(501) 378-2804 Fax

Oregon
Medicare B
Blue Cross/Blue Shield of
North Dakota
4510 13th Avenue, S.W.

Fargo, ND 58121
(701) 282-1100
(701) 282-1002 Fax

Pennsylvania
Medicare B
Medical Services Association of
Pennsylvania
P.O. Box 890065
Camp Hill, PA 17089-0065
(717) 763-3151
(717) 975-7045 Fax

Puerto Rico
Medicare B
Triple-S, Inc.
Box 363628
San Juan, PR 00936-3628
(787) 749-4080
(787) 749-4092 Fax

Rhode Island
Medicare B
Blue Cross/Blue Shield of
Rhode Island
444 Westminster Street
Providence, RI 02903-3279
(401) 459-1000
(401) 459-1709 Fax

South Carolina
Medicare B
Blue Cross/Blue Shield of
South Carolina
300 Arbor Lake Drive, Sutie
1300
Columbia, SC 29223
(803) 735-1034
(803) 691-2188 Fax

South Dakota
Medicare B
Blue Cross/Blue Shield of
North Dakota
4510 13th Avenue, S.W.
Fargo, ND 58121
(701) 282-1100
(701) 282-1002 Fax

Tennessee
Medicare B
Connecticut General Life
Insurance Company (CGLIC)
Hartford, CT 06152
(615) 782-4576
(615) 244-6242 Fax

Texas
Medicare B
Blue Cross/Blue Shield of
Texas, Inc.
901 South Central Expressway
Richardson, TX 75080
(214) 766-6900
(214) 766-7612 Fax

Utah
Medicare B
Blue Cross/Shield of Utah
1455 Parley's Way
P.O. Box 30270
Salt Lake City, UT 84130
(801) 487-6441
(801) 481-6994 Fax

Vermont
Medicare B
Blue Cross/Blue Shield of
Massachusetts
100 Summer Street

Boston, MA 02110
(617) 956-3445
(617) 350-4555 Fax

Virgin Islands
Medicare
Seguros De Servicio De Salud
De Puerto Rico
Call Box 71391
San Juan, Puerto Rico, 00936

Virginia
Medicare B
Metrahealth Insurance
Company
450 Columbus
Boulevard—5GB
P.O. Box 15045
Hartford, CT 06115-0450
(860) 702-6668
(860) 702-6587 Fax

Washington
Medicare B
Blue Cross/Blue Shield of
North Dakota
4510 13th Avenue, S.W.
Fargo, ND 58121
(701) 282-1100
(701) 282-1002 Fax

West Virginia
Medicare B
Nationwide Mutual Insurance
Company
P.O. Box 16788
Columbus, OH 43216
(614) 249-7111
(614) 249-3732 Fax

Wisconsin
Medicare B
Wisconsin Physicians' Service
Insurance Corp.
P.O. Box 1787
Madison, WI 53701
(608) 221-4711
(608) 223-3614 Fax

Wyoming
Medicare B
Blue Cross/Blue Shield of
North Dakota
4510 13th Avenue, S.W.
Fargo, ND 58121
(701) 282-1100
(701) 282-1002 Fax

APPENDIX 2

Vignettes for New Psychotherapy Codes

Office or Other Outpatient Facility

Insight-Oriented, Behavior-Modifying, and/or Supportive Psychotherapy

New CPT code: 90804
CPT code descriptor: Individual psychotherapy, insight oriented, behavior modifying, and/or supportive, in an office or outpatient facility, approximately 20–30 minutes face-to-face with the patient.

    These clinical examples have not been subjected to a uniform validation process by the American Medical Association, and do not appear in the American Medical Association's 1998 *Physicians' Current Procedural Terminology* or *Clinical Examples Supplement.*

Typical patient/service:

- Approximately 20–30 minutes psychotherapy with an obsessive-compulsive 29-year-old woman, last seen 6 weeks ago, who begins to pull out her hair uncontrollably after she is fired from her job.
- Approximately 20–30 minutes psychotherapy with a 12-year-old boy who has major depression, single episode, and who has been seen in outpatient psychotherapy for 9 months and is stable.

New CPT code: **90805**
CPT code descriptor: Individual psychotherapy, insight oriented, behavior modifying, and/or supportive, in an office or outpatient facility, approximately 20–30 minutes face-to-face with the patient, with medical evaluation and management services.

Typical patient/service:

- Approximately 20–30 minutes psychotherapy with an obsessive-compulsive 29-year-old woman, last seen 6 weeks ago, who takes clomipramine and begins to pull out her hair uncontrollably after she is fired from her job. Consider strategy for augmenting medication regimen.
- Approximately 20–30 minutes psychotherapy with a 12-year-old boy who has major depression, single episode, and who has been seen in outpatient psychotherapy for 9 months and is stable. Patient's condition improves with antidepressants. Patient asks about stopping medications. Consider altering medication and evaluating compliance.

New CPT code: **90806**
CPT code descriptor: Individual psychotherapy, insight oriented, behavior modifying, and/or supportive, in an office or outpatient facility, approximately 45–50 minutes face-to-face with the patient.

Typical patient/service:

- Approximately 45–50 minutes individual psychotherapy in office with a 52-year-old woman who has dysthymic disorder and a dependent personality disorder treated with insight-oriented therapy.
- Approximately 45–50 minutes individual psychotherapy in office with a 16-year-old girl who has panic disorder treated with cognitive-behavior therapy.

New CPT code: **90807**
CPT code descriptor: Individual psychotherapy, insight oriented, behavior modifying, and/or supportive, in an office or outpatient facility, approximately 45–50 minutes face-to-face with the patient, with medical evaluation and management services.

Typical patient/service:

- Approximately 45–50 minutes individual psychotherapy in office with a 72-year-old woman who has a major depressive disorder, recurrent COPD, congestive heart failure, and who takes antidepressant medication. Consider comorbid medical diagnoses, interaction of medication, and laboratory screening and interpretation.
- Approximately 45–50 minutes individual psychotherapy in office with a 16-year-old girl who has panic disorder treated with cognitive-behavior therapy, a tricyclic, and alprazolam.

New CPT code: **90808**

CPT code descriptor: Individual psychotherapy, insight oriented, behavior modifying, and/or supportive, in an office or outpatient facility, approximately 75–80 minutes face-to-face with the patient.

Typical patient/service:

- Approximately 75–80 minutes individual psychotherapy with established patient, a 41-year-old man with post-traumatic stress disorder. He has complaints of sudden reoccurrence of insomnia, anxiety attacks with uncontrolled shaking, anger outbursts, and flashbacks. He feels overwhelmed and unable to meet the needs of either his children or his job.
- Approximately 75–80 minutes individual psychotherapy in office with a 17-year-old boy who discloses for the first time his worries that he is homosexual and expresses suicidal ideation.

New CPT code: **90809**

CPT code descriptor: Individual psychotherapy, insight oriented, behavior modifying, and/or supportive, in an office or outpatient facility, approximately 75–80 minutes face-to-face with the patient, with medical evaluation and management services.

Typical patient/service:

- Approximately 75–80 minutes individual psychotherapy with established patient, a 35-year-old man with bipolar I disorder who is on divalproex and an SSRI. He reports the sudden onset of irritability, flights of ideas, and sleeplessness. Obtain divalproex level and discontinue SSRI.

- Approximately 75–80 minutes individual psychotherapy in office with a 17-year-old girl recently diagnosed as having schizophrenia. She has stopped taking her medication, has become increasingly paranoid, and has verbally threatened her family. Evaluate for comorbid medical illness; laboratory screening and interpretation; consider change in medication.

Interactive Psychotherapy

New CPT code: **90810**

CPT code descriptor: Individual psychotherapy, interactive, using play equipment, physical devices, language interpreter, or other mechanisms of nonverbal communication, in an office or outpatient facility, approximately 20–30 minutes face-to-face with the patient.

Typical patient/service:

- Approximately 20–30 minutes interactive psychotherapy with a 6-year-old boy who has oppositional defiant disorder and whose tantrums and stubborn refusal to follow instructions began after his mother's remarriage.

New CPT code: **90811**

CPT code descriptor: Individual psychotherapy, interactive, using play equipment, physical devices, language interpreter, or other mechanisms of nonverbal communication, in an office or outpatient facility, approximately 20–30 minutes face-to-face with the patient, with medical evaluation and management services.

Typical patient/service:

- Approximately 20–30 minutes interactive psychotherapy with a 9-year-old boy who has attention-deficit/hyperactivity disorder and at times refuses to take his stimulant medication and whose teachers have not reported a robust response to the medication.

New CPT code: **90812**
CPT code descriptor: Individual psychotherapy, interactive, using play equipment, physical devices, language interpreter, or other mechanisms of nonverbal communication, in an office or outpatient facility, approximately 45–50 minutes face-to-face with the patient.

Typical patient/service:

- Approximately 45–50 minutes interactive psychotherapy with a 6-year-old girl who has a history of separation anxiety disorder. Although she is sleeping better, she is still frightened at school and other locations away from her parents.

New CPT code: **90813**
CPT code descriptor: Individual psychotherapy, interactive, using play equipment, physical devices, language interpreter, or other mechanisms of nonverbal communication, in an office or outpatient facility, approximately 45–50 minutes face-to-face with the patient, with medical evaluation and management services.

Typical patient/service:

- Approximately 45–50 minutes interactive psychotherapy with an 8-year-old girl who has a history of separation anxiety disorder and generalized anxiety disorder and is seen for monthly medication management and short-term psychotherapy. She requires assistance with a scheduled surgical procedure that necessitates general anesthesia. She requires face-to-face time and clay materials to enact the hospital admission and surgical procedure. Evaluation of potential interaction between psychotropic medications and anesthesia also required.

New CPT code: **90814**
CPT code descriptor: Individual psychotherapy, interactive, using play equipment, physical devices, language interpreter, or other mechanisms of nonverbal communication, in an office or outpatient facility, approximately 75–80 minutes face-to-face with the patient.

Typical patient/service:

- Approximately 75–80 minutes interactive psychotherapy with an 8-year-old boy who has a history of sexual abuse and persistent problems with sleeping, eating, and sustaining relationships.

New CPT code: **90815**
CPT code descriptor: Individual psychotherapy, interactive, using play equipment, physical devices, language interpreter, or other mechanisms of nonverbal communication, in an office or outpatient facility, approximately 75–80 minutes face-to-face with the patient, with medical evaluation and management services.

Typical patient/service:

- Approximately 75–80 minutes interactive psychotherapy with an 8-year-old boy who has a history of sexual abuse and persistent problems with sleeping, eating, and sustaining relationships. Medication to manage anxiety, distractibility, and mood disturbance has been only modestly helpful.

Inpatient Hospital, Partial Hospital, or Residential Care Facility

Insight-Oriented, Behavior-Modifying, and/or Supportive Psychotherapy

New CPT code: **90816**

CPT code descriptor: Individual psychotherapy, insight oriented, behavior modifying, and/or supportive, in an inpatient hospital, partial hospitalization, or residential care setting, approximately 20–30 minutes face-to-face with the patient.

Typical patient/service:

- Approximately 20–30 minutes psychotherapy in hospital on day before discharge for a 24-year-old woman with borderline personality disorder.
- Approximately 20–30 minutes individual psychotherapy in residential treatment center with a 14-year-old boy who has conduct disorder and who periodically requires seclusion for aggression.

New CPT code: **90817**

CPT code descriptor: Individual psychotherapy, insight oriented, behavior modifying, and/or supportive, in an inpatient hospital, partial hospitalization, or residential care setting, approximately 20–30 minutes face-to-face with the patient, with medical evaluation and management services.

Typical patient/service:

- Approximately 20–30 minutes individual psychotherapy in nursing home with an 85-year-old woman who has carcinoma metastatic to lung and adjustment disorder with depression. Antidepressant medication prescribed.

- Approximately 20–30 minutes individual psychotherapy in residential treatment center with a 14-year-old boy who has schizophrenia, who takes an atypical neuroleptic requiring laboratory monitoring, and who periodically requires seclusion for aggression.

New CPT code: **90818**
CPT code descriptor: Individual psychotherapy, insight oriented, behavior modifying, and/or supportive, in an inpatient hospital, partial hospitalization, or residential care setting, approximately 45–50 minutes face-to-face with the patient.

Typical patient/service:

- Approximately 45–50 minutes individual psychotherapy in hospital with a 35-year-old woman who has postpartum depression and is about to be discharged.
- Approximately 45–50 minutes individual psychotherapy in hospital with a 15-year-old boy hospitalized for detoxification and prepared for transfer to partial hospitalization program.

New CPT code: **90819**
CPT code descriptor: Individual psychotherapy, insight oriented, behavior modifying, and/or supportive, in an inpatient hospital, partial hospitalization, or residential care setting, approximately 45–50 minutes face-to-face with the patient, with medical evaluation and management services.

Typical patient/service:

- Approximately 45–50 minutes individual psychotherapy in hospital with a 65-year-old woman who has major depression, is unresponsive to antidepressant medication, and is being prepared for electroconvulsive therapy. Laboratory screening and interpretation; consider underlying comorbid medical diagnosis.

- Approximately 45–50 minutes individual psychotherapy in hospital with a 16-year-old girl hospitalized for acute psychosis secondary to abuse of diet pills. Laboratory screening and interpretation and medication evaluation required.

New CPT code: **90821**
CPT code descriptor: Individual psychotherapy, insight oriented, behavior modifying, and/or supportive, in an inpatient hospital, partial hospitalization, or residential care setting, approximately 75–80 minutes face-to-face with the patient.

Typical patient/service:

- Approximately 75–80 minutes psychotherapy in nursing home with a 78-year-old woman who has had an altercation with another patient.
- Approximately 75–80 minutes psychotherapy in partial hospitalization setting with a 15-year-old girl who has anorexia nervosa and struggles with continued relapses. She has had a 4-lb weight loss in the past week.

New CPT code: **90822**
CPT code descriptor: Individual psychotherapy, insight oriented, behavior modifying, and/or supportive, in an inpatient hospital, partial hospitalization, or residential care setting, approximately 75–80 minutes face-to-face with the patient, with medical evaluation and management services.

Typical patient/service:

- Approximately 75–80 minutes psychotherapy in hospital with a 68-year-old woman who has bipolar disorder and has attempted suicide. Patient will be placed in congregate living facility upon discharge. Patient has many questions about her medication and its management. Requires laboratory screening and interpretation. Evaluate medication for potential side effects and drug interactions.

- Approximately 75–80 minutes psychotherapy in partial hospitalization setting with a 17-year-old girl who has schizophrenia. She has begun abusing alcohol. Laboratory screening and interpretation and medication evaluation required.

Interactive Psychotherapy

New CPT code: **90823**
CPT code descriptor: Individual psychotherapy, interactive, using play equipment, physical devices, language interpreter, or other mechanisms of nonverbal communication, in an inpatient hospital, partial hospitalization, or residential care setting, approximately 20–30 minutes face-to-face with the patient.

Typical patient/service:

- Approximately 20–30 minutes interactive psychotherapy with an 8-year-old girl with mild mental retardation who was hospitalized because of violent outbursts. Her parents state they are no longer able to control her.

New CPT code: **90824**
CPT code descriptor: Individual psychotherapy, interactive, using play equipment, physical devices, language interpreter, or other mechanisms of nonverbal communication, in an inpatient hospital, partial hospitalization, or residential care setting, approximately 20–30 minutes face-to-face with the patient, with medical evaluation and management services.

Typical patient/service:

- Approximately 20–30 minutes interactive psychotherapy with an 8-year-old girl with mild mental retardation and a seizure disorder who was hospitalized because of violent outbursts. Reevaluation of seizure medication required.

New CPT code: **90826**
CPT code descriptor: Individual psychotherapy, interactive, using play equipment, physical devices, language interpreter, or other mechanisms of nonverbal communication, in an inpatient hospital, partial hospitalization, or residential care setting, approximately 45–50 minutes face-to-face with the patient.

Typical patient/service:

- Approximately 45–50 minutes interactive psychotherapy with a 7-year-old girl who is combative and making multiple superficial cuts on her arm. She is hospitalized for self-destructive behavior. Because of a history of physical and sexual abuse, she has been removed from her home and placed in the custody of child protective services.

New CPT code: **90827**
CPT code descriptor: Individual psychotherapy, interactive, using play equipment, physical devices, language interpreter, or other mechanisms of nonverbal communication, in an inpatient hospital, partial hospitalization, or residential care setting, approximately 45–50 minutes face-to-face with the patient, with medical evaluation and management services.

Typical patient/service:

• Approximately 45–50 minutes interactive psychotherapy with an 8-year-old boy who is self-destructive and aggressive and has bipolar disorder. He no longer can be managed in a partial hospital program and therefore requires residential treatment. His predominant mood is anger, and he refuses to discuss the traumas and losses he has endured. He has not yet responded to a combination of mood stabilizer and antidepressant medication. Laboratory screening and interpretation and medication management.

New CPT code: **90828**
CPT code descriptor: Individual psychotherapy, interactive, using play equipment, physical devices, language interpreter, or other mechanisms of nonverbal communication, in an inpatient hospital, partial hospitalization, or residential care setting, approximately 75–80 minutes face-to-face with the patient.

Typical patient/service:

• Approximately 75–80 minutes interactive psychotherapy with a 6-year-old boy hospitalized for violent behavior who has attacked another patient.

New CPT code: **90829**
CPT code descriptor: Individual psychotherapy, interactive, using play equipment, physical devices, language interpreter, or other mechanisms of nonverbal communication, in an inpatient hospital, partial hospitalization, or residential care setting, approximately 75–80 minutes face-to-face with the patient, with medical evaluation and management services.

Typical patient/service:

- Approximately 75–80 minutes interactive psychotherapy with a 70-year-old man who has been hospitalized for major depressive disorder and has had a cerebrovascular accident, with expressive aphasia and right hemiplegia. He also has developed unstable blood pressure while taking antidepressants. Consider comorbid medical diagnosis, medication evaluation, and antidepressant medications.

APPENDIX 3

Health Care Financing Administration Regional Offices

I n situations where the appropriate medical society liaison or a Medicare carrier is unable to provide adequate information, questions can be directed to the appropriate Health Care Financing Administration (HCFA) regional office. This listing provides addresses and phone numbers of the 10 HCFA regional offices across the country.

Region I—Boston
Connecticut, Maine,
Massachusetts, New Hampshire,
Rhode Island and Vermont
Associate Regional
Administrator
HCFA Program Operations
John F. Kennedy Federal
Building
Government Center
Room 2325
Boston, MA 02203-0033
(617) 565-1273

Region II—New York
New Jersey, New York, Puerto
Rico and Virgin Islands
Associate Regional
Administrator
HCFA Program Operations
26 Federal Plaza, Room 3811
New York, NY 10278-0063
(212) 264-8517

Region III—Philadelphia
Delaware, District of Columbia,
Maryland, Pennsylvania,
Virginia and West Virginia
Associate Regional
Administrator
HCFA Program Operations
3535 Market Street
Room 3100
Philadelphia, PA 19104
(215) 596-6828

Region IV—Atlanta
Alabama, Florida, Georgia,
Kentucky, Mississippi, North
Carolina, South Carolina and

Tennessee
Associate Regional
Administrator HCFA Program
Operations
101 Marietta, Suite 701
Atlanta, GA 30323-2711
(404) 331-2548

Region V—Chicago
Indiana, Illinois, Michigan,
Minnesota, Ohio and Wisconsin
Associate Regional
Administrator
HCFA Program Operations
105 W. Adams Street
14th–16th Floors
Chicago, IL 60603-6201
(312) 353-9840

Region VI—Dallas
Arkansas, Louisiana, Oklahoma,
New Mexico and Texas
Associate Regional
Administrator
HCFA Program Operations
1200 Main Tower Building
Suite 2000
Dallas, TX 75202-4305
(214) 767-6418

Region VII—Kansas City
Iowa, Kansas, Missouri and
Nebraska
Associate Regional
Administrator
HCFA Program Operations
New Federal Office Building
601 E. 12th Street, Room 235
Kansas City, MO 64106-2808
(816) 426-3539

Region VIII—Denver
Colorado, Montana, North Dakota, South Dakota, Wyoming, Utah
Associate Regional Administrator
HCFA Program Operations
1961 Stout Street, Room 1185
Denver, CO 80294-3538
(303) 844-6149, ext. 233

Region IX—San Francisco
Arizona, California, Nevada, Guam, Hawaii and American Samoa
Associate Regional Administrator HCFA Program Operations
75 Hawthorne Street
4th and 5th Floors
San Francisco, CA 94105-3903
(415) 744-3628

Region X—Seattle
Alaska, Idaho, Oregon and Washington
Associate Regional Administrator HCFA Program Operations
2201 Sixth Avenue, DPO-RX40
Seattle, WA 98121-2500
(206) 615-2345

References

Albaum-Feinstein AL: A health information manager's perspective: meeting the challenge of coding and documentation. Journal of Practical Psychiatry and Behavioral Health 2:146–150, 1996

American Medical Association: The CPT Process. Chicago, IL, American Medical Association, 1992a

American Medical Association: Physicians' Current Procedural Terminology 1992, 4th Edition. Chicago, IL, American Medical Association, 1992b

American Medical Association: Principles of Medical Documentation. Chicago, IL, American Medical Association, 1992c

American Medical Association: Medicare RBRVS: The Physicians' Guide. Chicago, IL, American Medical Association, 1996a

American Medical Association: Physicians' Current Procedural Terminology 1997. Chicago, IL, American Medical Association, 1996b

American Medical Association: Physicians' Current Procedural Terminology 1998. Chicago, IL, American Medical Association, 1997

American Psychiatric Association: Diagnostic and Statistical Manual of Mental Disorders, 4th Edition. Washington, DC, American Psychiatric Association, 1994

American Psychiatric Association, American Medical Association: Procedural Terminology for Psychiatrists. Washington, DC, American Psychiatric Association, 1980

CPT Assistant Newsletter, Documentation Guidelines, Vol 7, No 7, July 1997

Healthcare Financing Administration Common Procedure Coding System: Level II—National Codes. Washington, DC, US Government Printing Office, 1998

Hsiao W, Braun P: Refinement of the development of a resource-based relative value system for psychiatric services. National Institute of Mental Health contract, January 31, 1991

Index

*Page numbers printed in **boldface** type refer to
tables or figures.*

Added codes, 11, 13
AMA. *See* American Medical
    Association
American Academy of Child
    and Adolescent Psychiatry,
    2
American Hospital Association,
    6
American Medical Association
    (AMA), 2, 5–9, 78
    Department of Coding and
        Nomenclature, 13
    documentation guidelines
        of, 79–80
    input to development of
        Resource-Based
        Relative Value Scale,
        66–67
American Psychiatric
    Association (APA), 2, 6

Assembly of District
    Branches, 60
Committee on Managed
    Care, 60
EcoFacts, 58
Managed Care Help Line,
    62
Medicare Carrier Advisory
    Committee Network,
    113
Office of Economic Affairs
    and Practice
    Management, 13,
    111–113
*Procedural Terminology for
    Psychiatrists,* 2, 6
resources for handling
    problems with
    insurance companies,
    60, 62

American Psychiatric
Association (APA)
(*continued*)
Work Group on Codes and
Reimbursements, 2–3,
8, 60, 111
Work Group on the Harvard
Resource-Based
Relative Value Scale,
60
Amytal interview. *See* Sodium
amobarbital interview
Anesthesia services, 10,
23
Antitrust violations, 66
APA. *See* American Psychiatric
Association
Aphasia testing, 26
Appendix A of CPT, 10, 29
Appendix B of CPT, 11
Appendix C of CPT, 11
Appendix D of CPT, 11
Assembly of District Branches
(APA), 60
Attending physicians, 31–32,
71
guidelines for inpatient
progress note,
103–106
Audits of physician practices,
1, 21, 22, 102

Balanced Budget Act of 1997,
73
Barbiturates, 22
Behavior-modifying
psychotherapy, 17–19

inpatient hospital, partial
hospital, or residential
care facility, 130–133
office or other outpatient
facility, 123–127
Benzodiazepines, 22
Better Business Bureau, 57
Billing, fraudulent, 1, 17, 74
Biofeedback training, 23
Blue Cross/Blue Shield, 6, 66
Bundling of psychiatric
services, 4
Business aspects of practice, 1,
102

Carve-out programs, 52
Case management services, 36,
41, **46**, 47
Central nervous system
assessments/tests, 25–26
documentation guidelines
for, 97
Changed codes, 11, 13,
111–112
Chief complaint, 16, 38, 81, **82**
Children
interactive group
psychotherapy for, 21
interactive psychiatric
diagnostic interview
examination of, 17
Claims processing, 54–55,
109–110
Claims submission, 1, 61,
108–110
Clinical examples supplement
to CPT, 11

Clinical nurse specialists, 70

Clinical psychologists, 68–69, 71

Clinical social workers, 69, 71

Cognitive impairments, interactive psychiatric diagnostic interview examination of patients with, 17, 95–96

Commitment proceedings, 49

Committee on Managed Care (APA), 60

Communication impairments, interactive psychiatric diagnostic interview examination of patients with, 17, 95–96

Concurrent review of services, 52

Congressional Physician Payment Review Commission, 66

Consultation services, 36, **45**, 47–50, 95

Coordination of care, 41, 47, 48, 88

Coordination of services with agencies, employers, or institutions, 23–24

Council of Economic Affairs, 2

Counseling, 40–41, 47, 88

Court testimony, 28

CPT. *See Physicians' Current Procedural Terminology*

Data bases of physician charging activity, 102

Deleted codes, 11, 12

Department of Coding and Nomenclature (AMA), 13

Desensitization therapy, 24

Developmental testing, 26

Diagnosis-related groups (DRGs), 66

Diagnostic and Statistical Manual of Mental Disorders (DSM-IV), 101

Diagnostic evaluation
codes for, 16–17, 31
documentation guidelines for, 95–96
elements of, 95
interactive psychiatric diagnostic interview examination, 17, 95–96

Disputes over third-party payments, 58–62, 112

Documenting insurance company contacts, 58

Documenting services, 1–3, 77–100, 103–107
American Medical Association's principles for, 79–80
guidelines for evaluation and management services, 78, 80–94
examination, 81, **86–88**
history taking, 81, **82–85**
medical decision making, 81, 83, **89–93**
proposed changes to, 88–89, 94

Documenting services
(*continued*)
  guidelines for evaluation
    and management
    services (*continued*)
    sources of, 80
    time, 83, **94**
    timeline for
      implementation of,
      80, 88
  guidelines for psychiatric
    diagnostic and
    therapeutic
    procedures, 78, 94–97
  general clinical
    psychiatric
    diagnostic or
    evaluative
    procedure, 95
  general guidelines for
    therapeutic
    procedures, 96
  individual psychotherapy,
    97
  inpatient attending
    progress note,
    103–106
  interactive group
    psychotherapy,
    97
  interactive psychiatric
    diagnostic interview
    examination,
    95–96
  lack of standardization of,
    94–95
  narcosynthesis, 97

  neurocognitive, mental
    status, and speech
    testing, 97
  outpatient progress note,
    106–107
  psychoanalysis, 97
for Medicare
  reimbursement,
  78
outpatient and inpatient
  services, 78–79
questions and answers
  about, 97–100
reasons for, 77–78
tailoring record-keeping
  system for, 97–98
Domiciliary, rest home, or
  custodial care services, 36,
  45–46, 47
DRGs. *See* Diagnosis-related
  groups
DSM-IV. *See Diagnostic and
  Statistical Manual of Mental
  Disorders*

EcoFacts, 58
Electroconvulsive therapy, 16,
  22–23, 30
E/M services. *See*Evaluation
  and management services
Emergency services, 36, 37,
  45, 47
Environmental interventions
  with agencies, employers,
  or institutions,
  23–24
Errors in coding, 1

Ethics of informing patients about problems with insurance companies, 62

Evaluation and management (E/M) services, 2, 4, 10, 12, 14–16, 35–50
  categories and definitions of, 36–37
  codes most likely to be used by psychiatrists, 44, **45–46**, 47–48
  components of level of, 37–43
    coordination of care, 41, 47, 48
    counseling, 40–41, 47
    examination, 39, 46, 81, **86–88**
    history taking, 38, 46, 81, **82–85**
    medical decision making, 39–40, **40**, 47, 81, 83, **89–93**
    nature of presenting problem, 41–42
    time, 42–43, 47, 49, 83, **94**
  documentation guidelines for, 78, 80–94, **82–94** (*See also* Documenting services)
  generic nature of, 35
  inpatient, 31–32, 42–43
  listing of, 36
  Medicare teaching-physician rule for, 72–73

  modifier for prolonged services, 30
  for new and established patients, 36, 37, **45–46**
  notations for, 36
  psychotherapy with and without, 17–19
  questions and answers about, 48–50
  selecting codes for, 35–36, 108
  selecting level of, 44–48
Examination of patient
  documentation guidelines for, 81, **86–88**, 89, 98
  levels of service for, 39, 46, **88**
  psychiatric, 81, **86–87**
  using patient checklist for, 98
Explaining results of tests and examinations to family or other responsible persons, 24–25

Family history, 16, 38, 81, **83**, **85**, 100
Family psychotherapy, 20, 96
  conjoint (with patient present), 20, 96
  multiple-family group psychotherapy, 20, 96
  without patient present, 20
Federal Trade Commission, 66
Fee-for-service, 64
Fraudulent practices, 1, 17, 74

Geographic differences in
     practice costs, 67
Graduate medical education
     (GME), 72–73
Group psychotherapy, 20–21,
     96
     interactive, 21, 96, 97
     multiple-family, 20

Halstead-Reitan test battery,
     26
HCFA. *See* Health Care
     Financing Administration
Health care cost escalation,
     52–53
Health Care Financing
     Administration (HCFA), 1,
     3, 6, 9, 22, 66, 68, 78, 102,
     115
     Common Procedure Coding
          System, 68
     regional offices of, 137–139
Health Insurance Association
     of America, 6
Health insurance companies, 3,
     6, 14, 51–62
     alternative products of,
          52–53
     changes in health system
          affecting, 52–53
     claims processing by,
          54–55, 109–110
     developing and maintaining
          relationships with,
          56–58
     documentation of services
          required by, 78

documenting contacts with,
     58
filing record of mode of
     practice with,
     57–58
handling disputes with,
     58–62, 112
history of, 51–52
ideal relationship among
     patient, physician,
     and, 55–56
informing patients about
     problems with, 62
organization and
     management of,
     53–54
questions and answers
     about, 61–62
regulation and oversight of,
     55, 61
sources of information
     about, 58, 59
submitting claims to, 1, 61,
     108–110
Health maintenance
     organizations (HMOs), 52,
     53, 62
History of present illness
     (HPI), 16, 38, **82, 84,** 89,
     98–99
History taking, 16, 95
     chief complaint, 16, 38, 81,
          82
     construction of patient's
          history, **82–83**
     data collection methods for,
          99–100

documentation guidelines
for, 81, **82–85**, 88–89,
98–100
history of present illness,
16, 38, **82**, **84**, 89,
98–99
levels of service for, 38, 46,
84–85
past, family, and social
history, 16, 38, 81, **83**,
85, 89
review of systems, 16, 38,
81, **82**, **84–85**, 89,
98–99
HMOs. *See* Health maintenance
organizations
Home services, 36, **46**, 47
Hospital record evaluation, 24
Hospitalization. *See* Inpatient
services
HPI. *See* History of present
illness
Hypnotherapy, 23

ICD-9-CM. *See International
Classification of Diseases,
Ninth Revision, Clinical
Modification*
Identifying and recording of all
services provided,
102–103
"Incident to" services, 70–71
Index of CPT, 11–12
Information technologies,
101–102
Injections, Medicare payment
policy for, 68, **69**

Inpatient services, 12, 13,
15–16
documentation of, 79
guidelines for inpatient
attending progress
note, 103–106
evaluation and
management
services, 36, 42–43,
45, 47–50
Medicare teaching-physician
rules and, 71–73
provided by attending
psychiatrist, 31–32
psychiatric diagnostic
interview
examination, 15–17,
31
psychotherapy, 19, 31,
130–136
interactive, 133–136
time spent providing,
42–43
Insight-oriented
psychotherapy, 17–19
inpatient hospital, partial
hospital, or residential
care facility, 130–133
office or other outpatient
facility, 123–127
Interactive diagnostic interview
examination, 17
documentation guidelines
for, 95–96
Interactive psychotherapy,
17–19
group, 21, 96, 97

Interactive psychotherapy
(*continued*)
inpatient hospital, partial
hospital, or residential
care facility,
133–136
office or other outpatient
facility, 127–129
*International Classification of
Diseases, Ninth Revision,
Clinical Modification*
(ICD-9-CM), 80, 101
Introductory section of CPT,
10

Laboratory services, 10, 16
specimen handling and
transfer for, 27
Legal counsel regarding
problems with insurance
companies, 60–61
Liability insurance,
professional, 67
Light therapy, 27
Luria test battery, 26

Managed Care Help Line
(APA), 62
Managed care organizations, 1,
3–4, 52–53, 62, 102
Mandated services, 30
Medicaid, 6, 52
Medical decision making,
39–40, 47
amount and/or complexity
of data to be reviewed,
91

criteria leading to level of,
39–40, **40**, **89**
definition of, 39
documentation guidelines
for, 81, 83, 89, **89–93**,
94
number of diagnoses or
management options,
90
risk of complications
and/or morbidity
or mortality,
92–93
Medical services, 10
Medical testimony, 28
Medicare, 3, 6, 9, 32, 52,
63–75
basic payment mechanism
of, 64, 74–75
participating approved
charges,
nonparticipating
approved charges,
and limiting
charges, 64, 74
patient copayments, 64,
74–75
benefits of participation
versus
nonparticipation in,
65, 74
documentation of services
required under,
78
establishment of, 63
listing of Part B carriers,
115–122

Medicare RBRVS: The Physicians' Guide, 67–68
Part A and Part B of, 63, 65–66
payment for nonphysicians, 68–71
clinical psychologists, 68–69
clinical social workers, 69
"incident to" services, 70–71
nurse practitioners and clinical nurse specialists, 70
physician assistants, 70
physician payment reform under, 65–68
private contracting under, 73
questions and answers about, 73–75, 112–113
reimbursement policies of
for evaluation and management services, 35, 72–73
for injections, 68, **69**
for inpatient services, 31–32
for psychiatric diagnostic interview examination, 16–17
resources for information about, 112–113
for telephone management, 68

teaching-physician rules under, 71–73
evaluation and management services, 72–73
general rule, 71–72
Medicare Carrier Advisory Committee Network (APA), 113
Mental status examination, 16, 22, 97
Minnesota Multiphasic Personality Inventory (MMPI), 26
Modifiers, 28–30
definition of, 28–29
explaining reason for use of, 29, 30
listing of, 10, 29
for mandated services, 30
notations about, 13, 16
for professional component, 30
for prolonged evaluation and management services, 30
for reduced services, 30
for services of clinical psychologists and clinical social workers, 71
for unusual procedural services, 29, 30, 33

Narcosynthesis, 22, 96
documentation guidelines for, 97

Nature of presenting problem, 41–42
Neurobehavioral status examination, 26
Neuropsychological testing, 26, 97
Notations, 13, 15–16
Nurse practitioners, 70
Nursing facility services, 32, 36, **45**, 47, 70

Office of Economic Affairs and Practice Management (APA), 13, 111–113
Office or other outpatient services
  documentation of, 78–79
    guidelines for outpatient progress note, 106–107
  evaluation and management services, **45**, 49
  provided at nonstandard times or places, 27
  psychotherapy, 18–19, 123–129
    interactive, 127–129
  time spent providing, 42
Orthotic devices, 27

Partial hospital services. *See also* Inpatient services
  psychotherapy, 19, 31, 130–136
PAs. *See* Physician assistants
Past history, 16, 38, 81, **83**, 85

Pathology, 10
Patient education materials, 28
Pharmacologic management, 4, 21–22, 32
  unbundling of psychotherapy from, 17, 22
Physician assistants (PAs), 70
Physician Payment Review Commission, 66
Physicians' Current Procedural Terminology (CPT), 2, 5–14, 80, 101
  changes to codes in, 12–13, 111–112
  codes deleted from, 11, 12
  CPT Advisory Committee, 7, 8
  CPT Editorial Panel, 2, 6, 7–9, 88, 111
  history of, 5–6
  organization of, 10–12
    Appendix A, 10, 29
    Appendix B, 11
    Appendix C, 11
    Appendix D, 11
    evaluation and management services, 10, 35–48
    index, 11–12
    introduction to manual, 10
    psychiatry subsection, 12, 15–31

sections on anesthesia, surgery, radiology, pathology and laboratory, and medicine, 10
purpose and goals of, 5
questions and answers about, 13–14
updating of, 7–9, 14
    criteria for, 8–9
    frequency of, 6
    keeping informed of changes due to, 111–112
    making request for, 7–9, 13
    process for, 7–9
Play therapy, 21
Point-of-service contracts, 52
PPOs. *See* Preferred provider organizations
Preauthorization for services, 52
Preferred provider organizations (PPOs), 52, 53
Preparation of reports, 25, 28
Preventive medicine services, 36, **46**, 47
Procedural coding, 1–4, 101–113
    bundling of psychiatric services for, 4
    documentation guidelines for, 77–100, 103–107
    effects of errors in, 1

for evaluation and management services, 35–50
health insurance companies and, 51–62, 108–110
importance of, 2, 101
Medicare and, 63–75
for psychiatric services, 15–31
questions and answers about, 111–113
recommendations for, 111
selecting codes for, 107–108
Professional component of procedure, 30
Professional liability insurance, 67
Progress notes, 103–107. *See also* Documenting services
    inpatient attending, 103–106
    outpatient, 106–107
Prosthetic devices, 27
Protective devices, 27
Psychiatric service codes, 15–33
    for central nervous system assessments/tests, 25–26, 97
    for evaluation and management services, 26, 35–48 (*See also* Evaluation and management services)
    modifiers for, 28–30
    notations for, 13, 15–16
    payer acceptance of, 32

Psychiatric service codes
     (*continued*)
  for psychiatric diagnostic or
       evaluative interview
       procedures, 12, 16–17
    documentation guidelines
       for, 95–96
  for psychiatric therapeutic
       procedures, 12, 17–25
    biofeedback training with
       psychotherapy, 23
    documentation guidelines
       for, 96–97
    electroconvulsive therapy,
       22–23
    environmental
       interventions with
       agencies, employers,
       or institutions,
       23–24
    explaining results of tests
       and examinations to
       family or other
       responsible persons,
       24–25
    hypnotherapy, 23
    pharmacologic
       management, 21–22
    preparing patient status
       reports, 25
    psychotherapy, 17–21
       (*See also*
       Psychotherapy)
    reviewing patient data,
       24
    sodium amobarbital
       interview, 22, 97

  unlisted services or
       procedures, 25,
       31
  questions and answers
       about, 31–33
  selection of, 107–108
  for special services and
       reports, 26–28
    emergency services, 27
    light therapy, 27
    medical devices, 27
    medical testimony, 28
    preparing reports, 28
    services provided at
       nonstandard times
       and places, 27
    specimen handling and
       transfer, 27
    supplies and materials,
       27–28
    travel expenses, 28
Psychiatry subsection of CPT,
     12, 15–25
Psychoanalysis, 19–20, 96
  documentation guidelines
     for, 97
Psychological testing, 25–26,
     97
Psychologists, 68–69, 71
Psychotherapy, 4, 12, 17–21,
     96
  biofeedback training with,
     23
  categories of codes for,
     17
  documentation guidelines
     for, 97

with and without evaluation and management services, 17–19
family, 20
group, 20–21
  interactive, 21, 97
  multiple-family, 20
in inpatient hospital, partial hospital, or residential care facility, 19, 31, 130–136
interactive, 17–19
  group, 21, 96, 97
  office or other outpatient, 127–129
Medicare copayment for, 64
in office or other outpatient facility, 18–19, 123–129
psychoanalysis, 19–20
site of service for, 18–19
telephone, 32–33
unbundling from other services, 17, 22
vignettes for new codes for, 123–136

Questions and answers
CPT, 13–14
documenting services, 97–100
evaluation and management services, 48–50
health insurance companies, 61–62, 112
Medicare, 73–75, 112–113

procedural coding, 111–113
psychiatric service codes, 31–33

Radiology services, 10
RBRVS. *See* Resource-Based Relative Value Scale
Reduced services, 30
Reimbursement, 1–4
documentation for, 1–3, 77–97
handling disputes over third-party payments, 58–62, 112
by health insurance companies, 51–61
managed care and, 52–53
under Medicare, 63–73
Related service codes, 4
Relative Value Units (RVUs), 3, 4, 31, 78
Report preparation, 25, 28
Residential care facilities, 32
psychotherapy in, 19, 31, 130–133
  interactive, 133–136
Residents' services, Medicare teaching-physician rules for, 71–73
Resource-Based Relative Value Scale (RBRVS), 1–4, 9, 63, 66–68
American Medical Association requirements for, 66–67
development of, 66

Resource-Based Relative
  Value Scale (RBRVS)
  (*continued*)
  importance of being familiar
    with, 73–74
  *Medicare RBRVS: The
    Physicians' Guide,*
    67–68
  RVS Update Committee, 9
  transition period for
    implementation of, 67
Retrospective review of
  services, 52
Review of patient's records, 24
Review of systems (ROS), 16,
  38, 81, **82, 84–85**, 89,
  98–99
Revised codes, 11, 13,
  111–112
Rorschach Test, 26
ROS. *See* Review of systems
RVS Update Committee
  (RUC), 9
RVUs. *See* Relative Value Units

Second opinions, 52
Selecting codes, 107–108
  for evaluation and
    management services,
    35–36, 108
Social history, 16, 38, 81, **83,
  85**, 100
Social workers, 69, 71
Sodium amobarbital interview,
  22, 96
  documentation guidelines
    for, 97

Special services and reports,
  26–28. *See also* Psychiatric
  service codes
Specimen handling and
  transfer, 27
Speech testing, 97
State insurance commissioners,
  55, 56, 61
State listing of Medicare Part B
  carriers, 116–122
Supplies, 27–28
Supportive psychotherapy,
  17–19
  inpatient hospital, partial
    hospital, or residential
    care facility, 130–133
  office or other outpatient
    facility, 123–127
Surgery, 10

Teaching-physician rules
  under Medicare, 71–73
  evaluation and management
    services, 72–73
  general rule, 71–72
Telephone services
  Medicare payment policy
    for, 68
  psychotherapy, 32–33
Testimony, medical, 28
Therapeutic procedures codes,
  12, 17–25. *See also*
  Psychiatric service codes
Time spent providing services,
  42–43, 47, 49
  choosing level based on, 43,
    94

documentation guidelines
for, 83, **94**
intraservice time, 42
pre- and postencounter
time, 42
unit/floor time, 42–43
Travel expenses, 28

Unbundling of psychiatric
services, 4, 17
Unlisted services or
procedures, 25, 31
Unusual procedural services
modifiers for, 29, 30
recurrent, 33
Utilization review, 52

Vignettes for new
psychotherapy codes,
123–136
inpatient hospital, partial
hospital, or residential
care facility, 130–136
insight-oriented,
behavior-modifying,
or supportive
psychotherapy,
130–133

interactive
psychotherapy,
133–136
office or other
outpatient facility,
123–129
insight-oriented,
behavior-
modifying, or
supportive
psychotherapy,
123–127
interactive
psychotherapy,
123–129

Wechsler Adult Intelligence
Scale—Revised (WAIS-R),
26
Work Group on Codes and
Reimbursements
(APA), 2–3, 8, 60,
111
Work Group on the
Harvard Resource-
Based Relative Value
Scale (APA), 60
Work site visits, 24